I0038366

Advances in Biobanking Practice Through Public and Private Collaborations

Edited by

Elena Salvaterra

Founder and Director of Areteva, Sherwood House, 7 Gregory Boulevard, Nottingham, Nottinghamshire, NG7 6LB

&

Julie Corfield

Coordinator Scientific Projects and Regulatory Affairs, Exem Italia s.r.l., Italy; ISBER Science and Policy Committee Advisor (US), ESBB Founder Member (EU), Organ Preservation Alliance Member (US)

BENTHAM SCIENCE PUBLISHERS LTD.
End User License Agreement (for non-institutional, personal use)

This is an agreement between you and Bentham Science Publishers Ltd. Please read this License Agreement carefully before using the ebook/echapter/ejournal (**"Work"**). Your use of the Work constitutes your agreement to the terms and conditions set forth in this License Agreement. If you do not agree to these terms and conditions then you should not use the Work.

Bentham Science Publishers agrees to grant you a non-exclusive, non-transferable limited license to use the Work subject to and in accordance with the following terms and conditions. This License Agreement is for non-library, personal use only. For a library / institutional / multi user license in respect of the Work, please contact: permission@benthamscience.org.

Usage Rules:

1. All rights reserved: The Work is the subject of copyright and Bentham Science Publishers either owns the Work (and the copyright in it) or is licensed to distribute the Work. You shall not copy, reproduce, modify, remove, delete, augment, add to, publish, transmit, sell, resell, create derivative works from, or in any way exploit the Work or make the Work available for others to do any of the same, in any form or by any means, in whole or in part, in each case without the prior written permission of Bentham Science Publishers, unless stated otherwise in this License Agreement.
2. You may download a copy of the Work on one occasion to one personal computer (including tablet, laptop, desktop, or other such devices). You may make one back-up copy of the Work to avoid losing it. The following DRM (Digital Rights Management) policy may also be applicable to the Work at Bentham Science Publishers' election, acting in its sole discretion:

• 25 'copy' commands can be executed every 7 days in respect of the Work. The text selected for copying cannot extend to more than a single page. Each time a text 'copy' command is executed, irrespective of whether the text selection is made from within one page or from separate pages, it will be considered as a separate / individual 'copy' command.
• 25 pages only from the Work can be printed every 7 days.

3. The unauthorised use or distribution of copyrighted or other proprietary content is illegal and could subject you to liability for substantial money damages. You will be liable for any damage resulting from your misuse of the Work or any violation of this License Agreement, including any infringement by you of copyrights or proprietary rights.

Disclaimer:

Bentham Science Publishers does not guarantee that the information in the Work is error-free, or warrant that it will meet your requirements or that access to the Work will be uninterrupted or error-free. The Work is provided "as is" without warranty of any kind, either express or implied or statutory, including, without limitation, implied warranties of merchantability and fitness for a particular purpose. The entire risk as to the results and performance of the Work is assumed by you. No responsibility is assumed by Bentham Science Publishers, its staff, editors and/or authors for any injury and/or damage to persons or property as a matter of products liability, negligence or otherwise, or from any use or operation of any methods, products instruction, advertisements or ideas contained in the Work.

Limitation of Liability:

In no event will Bentham Science Publishers, its staff, editors and/or authors, be liable for any damages, including, without limitation, special, incidental and/or consequential damages and/or damages for lost data and/or profits arising out of (whether directly or indirectly) the use or inability to use the Work. The entire liability of Bentham Science Publishers shall be limited to the amount actually paid by you for the Work.

General:

1. Any dispute or claim arising out of or in connection with this License Agreement or the Work (including non-contractual disputes or claims) will be governed by and construed in accordance with the laws of the U.A.E. as applied in the Emirate of Dubai. Each party agrees that the courts of the Emirate of Dubai shall have exclusive jurisdiction to settle any dispute or claim arising out of or in connection with this License Agreement or the Work (including non-contractual disputes or claims).
2. Your rights under this License Agreement will automatically terminate without notice and without the need for a court order if at any point you breach any terms of this License Agreement. In no event will any delay or failure by Bentham Science Publishers in enforcing your compliance with this License Agreement constitute a waiver of any of its rights.
3. You acknowledge that you have read this License Agreement, and agree to be bound by its terms and conditions. To the extent that any other terms and conditions presented on any website of Bentham Science Publishers conflict with, or are inconsistent with, the terms and conditions set out in this License Agreement, you acknowledge that the terms and conditions set out in this License Agreement shall prevail.

Bentham Science Publishers Ltd.
Executive Suite Y - 2
PO Box 7917, Saif Zone
Sharjah, U.A.E.
Email: subscriptions@benthamscience.org

**BENTHAM
SCIENCE**

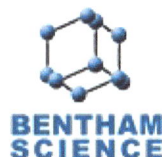

CONTENTS

FOREWORD 1

The present book addresses a significant gap in our collective knowledge on biobanking advancement through public-private partnerships. These partnerships are often alluded to in the peer-reviewed literature however one remains hard pressed to find and review a convincing, consistent body of evidence. The book moves quickly and effectively beyond a descriptive listing of the current landscape and sets as its core quest the aim of improvement. This improvement is multi-faceted: it can involve amongst others individual biobanks, collaborative projects, reference/national centers, qualitative standards, Intellectual Property (IP) issues, rights and obligations of stakeholders; all brought together for the common purpose of public and private benefit.

Over the past two decades the biobanking field has enjoyed a period of sustained investment, growth, wider scientific acceptance and development. Additionally, individual biobanks have benefited by support from very active, scientific community-driven societies, such as ISBER, the International Society for Biological and Environmental Repositories, and others. This has created a strong foundation for the regular exchange of experiences, the development of best practices and creation of educational tools with a global reach, especially as the biobanking field develops in Asia, Africa and south America. However, as the global financial crisis has developed into an enduring pressure for tighter cost control, expense justification and even cost retrieval, new operational models need to be considered for long-term sustainability in biobanking. This book investigates these alternative approaches which can operate in collaboration with the private sector yet without limiting their public benefit.

The editors have selected six distinct perspectives to provide a holistic approach in their subject. These are: Current practices; Quality management systems; Specimens quality; Rights and obligations of stakeholders; Collaboration models and Case studies. Sub-themes include the complementation and conflicts of different sectors and skill sets; the accreditation options and processes; the inherent trust in sample acquisition and processing, including biosafety. At the same time legal frameworks, different collaboration models and case studies are being brought together as a living corpus of evidence. It is indeed a very good collection of workable examples presented by some of the most respected scientific leaders in the field.

This book is an impressive and comprehensive study that moves beyond stereotypes that the biobanking field has often faced. It analyses why partnerships work and the future aspects that still need to be explored. Within the ISBER community there is the acute realization that private partners, commonly from the pharmaceutical industry, are often an essential component in addressing complex, healthcare related questions effectively and efficiently. The public –private partnerships have the potential to form a long-term, reliable infrastructure network enabling the discovery of new pharmaceutical agents, effective re-purposing of existing ones and preparedness in global health emergencies. I sincerely hope that more such examples will develop and strengthen in years to come, allaying public hesitation, and that a similar body of evidence will be developed in the not too distant future from our colleagues in Asia, Africa and south America.

Zisis Kozlakidis, Ph.D. AKC MBA FLS
ISBER 2016-17 President-elect
Chair, Centre of Excellence for Infectious Diseases BBMRI.uk
Division of Infection and Immunity
University College London
UK

FOREWORD 2

When walking the long way in the development of new products and methods to be used for patient treatment or diagnosis, medical translational research needs to be able to exchange knowledge and biomaterials in the public-private domain. Collaboration in this area is often indispensable for the final innovation of patient care. Funding institutions understand this need and increasingly try to stimulate this important domain where many exciting and interesting opportunities can be found. At the same time, it is also a difficult area to work with biomaterials as it means yet another boundary where you need to learn to deal with new often stricter rules with respect to ethics and regulatory issues. Yet this is certainly not the only aspect important for a smooth cooperation, also the quality of the samples are very crucial. Especially where reproducibility is concerned which can be a show stopper easily and unexpectedly encountered. Certainly the moment after the research process where a developed method or product needs to be validated for its intended use. In this step, one has to rely on the quality of the routine diagnostic samples which might be collected under very different pre-analytical conditions as the samples that were used in the discovery phase. The infrastructure of the biobank becomes very important. It should reflect or better yet make use of the existing routine diagnostic pathways. In addition, the quality of the diagnostic sample is in need for improvement to facilitate new products and methods more efficiently.

Of course there is an array of ways how the public and private partners can collaborate. Therefore, the editors have invited and selected the experts in their fields with much care to write chapters on:

- The importance, benefits and unique results that are obtained from the public private partnerships,
- Theoretical collaboration models and good examples of practical solutions and tips,
- How quality can contribute to the collaboration,
- The influence on legislation and ethics,
- Concrete examples of public-private collaborations based on local infrastructure synergies.

This logical line is also chosen to set up the book to become a consistent and structured overview of the complex domain of public private partnership. It consists of six interesting chapters, where each chapter starts with an abstract of the content. The field is an exciting and dynamic one with many opportunities for scientists from the academic setting and companies to find common grounds to synergistically grow in win-win environments.

Peter Riegman, Ph.D. AKC MBA FLS
Head Erasmus MC Tissue Bank,
PSI UMC Coordinator Erasmus MC,
ESBB Former President and ISBER Former President

PREFACE

The reflection on collaboration between public and private institutions in biobanking is crucial for making advances in this field.

Precision Medicine (PM), digitization and virtualization are quickly changing the biobanking landscape by asking for new models and concepts of synergies between public and private (or for profit) organizations.

However, this theme is currently under-analysis both in the literature and in scientific debates. The need for developing or improving collaborations between public and private institutions is recognized by several scholars but it still remains a niche topic in biobanking.

Furthermore, the reasons for developing public-private synergies (also called partnerships) are usually connected to biobank sustainability, on the public side, and to the acquisition of academic know how, on the private side.

This interpretation of the public-private-partnership (PPP) in biobanking seems to simplify the complexity of the issues related to public and private collaborations. It also seems to reduce the huge potentiality of promoting public-private synergies for biobanking advances and the related benefits for both public and private organizations working in this field.

Taking the above discussion into consideration, this ebook analyzes perspectives, methods and concrete ways to change the current models of collaboration between public and private organizations in order to improve biobanking practices.

The first chapter (Morente and colleagues) describes the state-of-the-art of public-private collaborations in biobanking on a global scale and it defines potential ways to improve these synergies. By highlighting that "the promotion of health" unconditionally should be the final goal of any partnership between public and private organization, Morente *et al.*, list several criteria to reconsider the current theories of PPP in biobanking.

Innovative approaches to public-private collaborations in biobanking are suggested by Lawlor and colleagues (chapter two). After an extensive analysis of "old" and current strategies of liaison in this realm, Lawlor *et al.*, recommend concrete models and methods of PPP to improve the biobanking practice.

The quality management system as a key aspect for public-private synergies in biobanking is the subject of chapter three. Bravo and colleagues extensively analyze the work of the technical committee "ISO T C 276 biotechnology" related to biotechnology standardization by focusing on biobanks and bioresources. The authors give a clear explanation of the role of ISO biotechnology standards to improve the quality of services for biobanks and to offer access to new markets for industries.

The description of quality standard criteria specifically tailored for tumor biobanks is provided by Bonizzi *et al.*, (chapter four). The authors report the standard requirements to be followed for processing samples and data in daily practice. These criteria are not different for public or private "partners". High level of quality is demanded by each organization for using the samples stored in the biobanks, regardless of the public or private nature of the inquiring institutions.

The access conditions to biobanks is the theme analyzed in chapter five by Verlinden and colleagues. After a deep analysis of the general legal framework governing biobanks at national (Belgium), European and international levels, Verlinden *et al.*, consider the access conditions to human biological samples and associated information.

Access conditions to samples and information stored in biobanks within the concrete model of the "HUB-BTB- 3CR" is the subject of chapter six. Di Donato *et al.*, describe the HUB-BTB-3CR which is a centralized organization for managing sample requests. This model enables public and private researchers to directly access the biobanks which are part of the hub. Although tailored for organizations operating in France, this prototype of public-private collaborations could be used in other countries with modifications as per requirements.

Moving from the theory to the practice, this ebook suggests an accessible analysis of the main issues related to public-private partnerships in biobanking. It considers apparently conflicting concepts, such as academia, industry, profit and solidarity illustrating that they are not necessarily in contrast when trust, transparency and reciprocity are the basis of public-private collaborations in biobanking.

Elena Salvaterra, JD, Ph.D. - Editor in Chief
Coordinator Scientific Projects and Regulatory Affairs
Exem Italia s.r.l., Italy; ISBER Science and Policy
Committee Advisor (US), ESBB Founder Member (EU)
Organ Preservation Alliance Member (US)
Italy

Julie Corfield
Founder and Director of Areteva, Sherwood House, 7
Gregory Boulevard, Nottingham, Nottinghamshire, NG7 6LB
UK

List of Contributors

Aldo Scarpa   ARC-Net, Applied Research on Cancer Center, University of Verona, Italy

Elena Bravo   Research Coordination and Support Service, Istituto Superiore di Sanità, Roma, Italy

Elena Salvaterra   ISBER Science and Policy Committee Advisor (US), ESBB Founder Member (EU), Organ Preservation Alliance Member (US), Coordinator Scientific Projects and Regulatory Affairs, Exem Italia s.r.l., Italy

Francisco de Luna   Spanish National Cancer Research Centre (CNIO), Calle Melchor Fernandez Almagro, 3. 28029 - Madrid, Spain

Giancarlo Pruneri   Director, Biobank for Translational Medicine Unit, European Institute of Oncology, Milano, Associate Professor in Pathology, University of Milano, School of Medicine, Italy

Giuseppina Bonizzi   Executive coordinator of Biobank for Translational Medicine Unit, European Oncology Institute (IEO), Milano, Italy

Herman Nys   Interfaculty Centre for Biomedical Ethics and Law, KU Leuven, KU Leuven, Belgium, Belgium

Isabelle Huys   Interfaculty Centre for Biomedical Ethics and Law, KU Leuven, KU Leuven, Belgium, Belgium

Jeanne-Hélène di Donato   1 impasse des Pinsons 31780 Castelginest, 3C-R, Biobank Consulting Company, France

Julie Corfield   Founder and Director of Areteva, Sherwood House, 7 Gregory Boulevard, Nottingham, Nottinghamshire, NG7 6LB, UK

Manuel M. Morente   Spanish National Cancer Research Centre (CNIO), Calle Melchor Fernandez Almagro, 3. 28029 - Madrid, Spain

Maria C. Marin   Spanish National Cancer Research Centre (CNIO), Calle Melchor Fernandez Almagro, 3. 28029 - Madrid, Spain

Mariarosaria Napolitano   Research Coordination and Support Service, Istituto Superiore di Sanità, Roma, Italy

Michiel Verlinden   Clinical Pharmacology and PharmacotherapyKU Leuven, Belgium

Nuria Ajenjo   Spanish National Cancer Research Centre (CNIO), Calle Melchor Fernandez Almagro, 3. 28029 - Madrid, Spain

Pascal Auré   BioTechBANK, 18 rue Proust, 49100 Angers, France

Rita T. Lawlor   ARC-Net, Applied Research on Cancer Center, University of Verona, Italy

CHAPTER 1

Public-Private Partnerships in Biobanking: Current Practices

Manuel M. Morente[*], **Francisco de Luna**, **Maria C. Marín** and **Nuria Ajenjo**

Spanish National Cancer Research Centre (CNIO), Spanish National Biobank Network ([**]), Madrid, Spain

Abstract: Public-private partnerships (PPPs) and relationships are essential to expedite the resolution of the challenges currently facing Medicine. Biobanking is not an island within biomedical research as a whole, and public–private partnerships in biobanking must therefore be considered in the global context of biomedical research.

PPPs are certainly desirable, since they offer benefits to both sides, create win-win situations and are extremely advantageous for the whole society, but they have their own limitations and frontiers.

The current chapter tries to introduce the general aspects of current PPP practices in biobanking, keeping in mind that the main objective should be the promotion of health rather than the sustainability of biobanks or benefits for industry.

Compliance with applicable legislation, mutual trust, transparency and open dialogue are the key components of such partnerships.

Keywords: Biobank management, Biobanking, Public-private partnership, Translational research.

INTRODUCTION: THE CHALLENGE OF PERSONALISED MEDICINE

Biospecimen science is a young and evolving discipline that arose from the paradigm shift induced by the great biotechnological advances that took place in the last decades of the 20th century and by the accessibility and knowledge of the human genome and its progressive application to healthcare in Personalised Medicine [1, 2]. These changes are triggering, indeed, a revolution in the study and understanding of more complex and multi-factorial diseases such as cancer,

[*] **Corresponding author Manuel M. Morente**: Spanish National Cancer Research Centre (CNIO), Calle Melchor Fernandez Almagro, 3. 28029 - Madrid, Spain; Tel: +34 91 732 80 00; E-mail: mmorente@cnio.es

[**] Spanish National Biobank Network is funded with public funds from the Instituto de Salud Carlos III, under the Health Strategic Actions 2010-2013 (RD09/0076) and 2014-2017 (PT13/0010)

Elena Salvaterra and Julie Corfield (Eds.)
All rights reserved-© 2017 Bentham Science Publishers

diabetes, and cardiovascular or neurodegenerative processes. This increased knowledge of the pathogenic bases of complex diseases is not merely of academic value, but it also has practical value that enables improvements in their prevention, diagnosis, prognostic evaluation and therapeutic approaches. Developing and evaluating novel therapies and diagnostic products requires access to rigorously designed and well-structured collections of biospecimens, and this places biobanking infrastructures in a critical position for the discovery, development and implementation of new drugs and products [3].

PUBLIC-PRIVATE RELATIONSHIPS: A NON-HOMOGENEOUS MODEL

Not only the academia and health care sectors are involved in this challenge, but also the industry [4], although their objectives do not always coincide. There are many nuances, but it can be said that health promotion and disease control are true goals in both sectors, although they are approached from different angles.

Before continuing this discussion, it is important to note that 'private' and 'public' have different meanings in different cultures and social models. Indeed, both terms have specific and differentiated connotations in, for instance, the United States of America, Europe, East Asia or emerging countries. Not only do these concepts have different meanings, but the private and public domains in the health care systems and biomedical research, including infrastructures such as biobanks, have a different weight. In addition, we can say the same about Europe as a whole, and about specific European countries, especially when an essential component of the discussion refers to health care systems. Domestic differences in public health care systems, in the development of funding of biomedical research by private charities, or in the dependence of research on public agencies are pivotal elements in private-public partnerships in biobanking.

Such differences also apply to biobanks. Thus, it has been said that "Commercial biobanks are attempting to position themselves as a, if not the, solution to problems that include a lack of public trust in researchers and lack of financial resources to support the prospective creation of collections that meet the highest scientific and ethical standards in the non-profit sector" [5]. This loss of trust is partially secondary to some examples of unethical practices that occurred in the past, and it has been suggested discomfort with the idea of gain from the mere transfer or exchange of human genetic material and information. However, this is not the actual situation in most of Europe, where academic research and researchers enjoy a high level of public trust, which is clearly higher than for industry-related research.

These differences and nuances cannot be discussed in depth in this chapter, and only general aspects can be included. Below we will focus on the Spanish social environment, which is characterised by a strong and very highly qualified public health system, little development of private charities funding biomedical research and hence a great dependence of research on public domestic or international (EU) agencies, and an increased presence of international pharmaceutical and biotechnology companies. The authors invite the readers to extend these thoughts to their own specific social environment.

THE PRIVATE AND THE PUBLIC SECTOR: TWO SECTORS WITH SPECIFIC OBJECTIVES, RESOURCES AND SKILLS

As was said above, both sectors (public and non-profit private institutions on the one hand and commercial institutions on the other) are involved and interested in the promotion of health, albeit with different and usually complementary objectives. While for the public sector, health promotion is the main objective, for the industrial sector, given its commercial character, profit is more important, although these are also important considerations in the academic setting. However, this basic difference in objectives is not an impediment to the need for both parties to establish efficient and effective ways of collaboration, especially in countries with advanced health systems of public character.

The private-industrial sector has the best capabilities for drug discovery and commercialization, biotechnology innovation, and the development of new products in order to facilitate biomedical research and public health. However, they usually have more difficulties accessing human samples and their associated clinical annotations, including adequate and long-term follow up, especially in those countries where the public sector is the most important agent of health care. On the other hand, the clinical sector (more frequently public in Europe) has more easy access to patients and healthy donors through hospital-based biobanks and is more dedicated to basic, translational and classic clinical research, but it is aware that it is not competent in the specific areas where industry has more expertise, resources and skills, and in fact almost only industry translates research into products [6].

However, the general landscape has changed in recent decades. Until the 1970s, academic research rarely worked on applied technologies, but the revolution of molecular genetics has enabled investigators to study, isolate and produce a large amount of molecules with medical properties. On this basis academia promotes a new era of relationships with industry, either directly or by using their own institutional offices for filing patents and licensing intellectual property to companies [6, 7].

These relationships certainly represent a great opportunity for solving health challenges and are overwhelmingly positive, but they are not exempt of problems. In order to abolish these problems some drastic decisions have been taken in the past. For instance, the director of the National Institutes of Health (NIH) prohibited in 2004 all corporate consulting activities and private investments by NIH researchers, who were obliged to stop all investments in health-related industries [8]. This ban represents an extreme, but in any case, these relationships need careful examination [7].

PPPS AND BIOBANK SUSTAINABILITY

It has been said that private-public partnerships (PPPs) are beneficial for the sustainability of biobanks, and this seems to be true, given the globally accepted fact of the impossibility of complete self-sustainability of general biobanks [2, 9], especially hospital-based banks and a wide range of disease-oriented banks.

European biobanks are subject to international and domestic legislation, which defines them as non-profit organizations even though a cost recovery policy is not only allowed but even advised [10]. However, most of specialists in biobanking consider self-sustainability exclusively based on cost recovery, as something close to a utopia [2].

As a rule, public biobank services to industry must be charged following a strict full-cost model [11], not only regarding the biobank-specific services provided to industry, but also in the context of a global partnership agreement.

THE STAKEHOLDERS

Focusing on human samples and hospital-based biobanks, and excluding pure genomic data repositories, there are four main groups of stakeholders to consider:

1. Public institutions, including national and international public funding agencies, researchers and research institutions.
2. Private- industrial institutions mainly represented by pharmaceutical industries, developers of biomarkers and diagnostic tools, biobank-related specific technology companies, and private service providers in biobanking.
3. Public biobanks and biobank networks.
4. Donors and society.

PUBLIC SECTOR AND NON-PROFIT AGENCIES

In some European countries, public agencies for research usually promote funding of collaborative projects through PPPs, where companies through soft credits or other incentives mainly obtain easier access to researchers of excellence working in the public sector. In such cooperative projects, if banked samples are needed, it would be good to prioritize the use of public biobanks in order to promote them and help them to be more sustainable, assuming a full-cost fee. For researchers this might provide a key opportunity to participate in new projects, obtain new ways of funding and create new strategic alliances for future projects.

In this sense, the initiative of the European Commission promoting large pan-European collaborative infrastructures (European Strategy Forum on Research Infrastructures – ESFRIs) and platforms based upon or open to public-private partnerships is applaudable [12].

INDUSTRY

Biomarker discovery and drug development programs rely on access to high-quality biospecimens. Therefore, biobanks, in particular tissue banks, are expected to become a key resource for the pharmaceutical industry [13]. Globally speaking, industry has been traditionally very reluctant to open PPPs. Fortunately, this is changing and currently research & development industries are more flexible and open to partnerships than in the past [14], although some aspects could be clearly improved. This change of mentality can be observed in the trend of some important pharmaceutical companies to externalise their R&D and innovation departments by closing contracts and establishing other ways of collaboration with universities and academic research centres, since this is a more efficient and cheap model.

Pharmaceutical companies play a special role. They are the main promoters of clinical trials and drug development and validation projects. Linked to these trials they usually not only recruit patients in terms of comprehensive clinical data, follow up, response, adverse effects, *etc.*, but they also obtain samples for pharmacogenomics and diagnostic evaluation. These samples, or their surplus, were almost never returned to the clinical archives or hospital-based biobanks, and most data obtained from these samples did not return to clinical records either. At least in the past and before current domestic and international legislative frameworks were in place, these samples were frequently used in other projects not included in the original donor consent. They apparently disappeared or were integrated into private and exclusive biobanks usually without control of the authorities, as opposed to what occurs in public biobanks. Furthermore, sometimes these samples were located in countries without specific legislation on biobanking.

It is fair to say, however, that this practice was not universal and did not apply to all pharmaceutical companies, hospitals, clinicians and biobanks. Some for-profit pharmaceutical companies, mainly some of the ones that are more prestigious and active in translational research, have assumed a leading role in assembling and managing these collections with the highest ethical and legal requisites [15], promoting well-organised banks based on the surplus of samples from clinical trials and other collaborative studies.

Some professionals and companies may claim that they own samples, but there is still no place for ownership of human tissue in the law [16], and this applies equally to individual researchers and institutions.

The case of **biotechnology companies**, mainly those who develop diagnostic and predictive markers and diagnostic products, is different. They are highly dependent on high quality samples and infrastructures in order to prove and validate their products, and they are therefore a great niche of opportunities for collaborations between private initiatives and public biobank holder institutions, with common benefits.

PUBLIC BIOBANKS AND BIOBANK NETWORKS

Public-hospital based biobanks can offer not only a large spectrum of disease-oriented samples and high quality associated information including follow-up, but they usually can also offer:

1. A great expertise,
2. High professionalization,
3. High quality due to established quality management systems and fulfilment of best practice guidelines [17 - 19],
4. Strict adherence to ethical and legal frameworks [20].

Collaborative Biobank Networks offer the most competitive service in public-private partnerships, mainly those with a federated model where each institution maintains its own collections but agrees to list them on a central shared database, and implement harmonised technical and ethic procedures . These networks offer the same advantages as isolated biobanks, plus the advantages of networking, including one-stop desks, centralised organization, harmonization, expert centres services, and scale advantages [21 - 23].

The importance of biobank networks has been emphasized by many authors and there are several major national and international networking initiatives worldwide [24]. This is even more relevant when rare diseases are the focus of the research, when molecular signatures consisting of multiple parameters have to be validated [25], or when researchers need samples from populations of different ethnic or regional origins.

DONORS

Finally, **donors** should also be considered in this stakeholders approach. They are willing to collaborate with public and/or non-profit biobanks, but they frequently express some degree of concern when they are informed that a private institution could use their samples, secondary products and data. It is a major challenge for biobank managers to guarantee privacy, and a common challenge for biobanks and industry to demonstrate the social benefits of such public-private partnership with no risks for donor privacy and rights [26].

It is all a matter of trust. Donors usually trust more in public biobanks and public research than in industry, but when patients have adequate information, donating the post-diagnosis surplus of surgically removed human tissue to biomedical research to be done in the commercial sector rather than donating to a public biobank is not a contentious issue [27]. An intense educational effort is needed, but this is not enough: transparency is essential and this also applies to the authorities. The authorities are obliged to improve transparency and implement control mechanisms when human subjects are used. Those controls should affect, at least to the same degree, public biobanks and industry-driven use of samples. This equality of social control (ethical and scientific review, external quality assurance, second use requisites, transparency, *etc.*) are not only an issue of a sense of justice among donors, but they are also essential for fair public-private partnerships.

BASES OF A FRUITFUL PPPS IN BIOBANKING

Industry must recognise the pivotal importance of the activities and services of public biobanks, and see biobanks as project partners and not only as sample providers. On the other hand, biobanks must accept the unique and indispensable role of industry in research and the promotion of public health, and be open to establishing transparent and stable public-private relationships.

Biobanks with a high degree of success regarding partnerships with industry are those who provide [28]:

1. Samples of high quality, including clinical data and certified quality of all processes involved [29].
2. Adequate communication channels in order to discuss and agree about required sample collecting, processing methods, production of derivatives, *etc.*
3. Flexibility and adaptability to industry requirements.
4. Confidentiality, which is critically important for industry.
5. Speed, because biotech business models are very time-sensitive.
6. Ancillary services if necessary, for instance case reviews by experienced

pathologists [30], tissue-microarray development, digitalization of slides, immune histochemical staining, and other techniques.

On the other hand, industries developing fluid and fruitful relationships with public biobanks are those who easily accept a number of principles:

1. Public institutions, including biobanks, have very strict and sometimes restrictive obligations and legal requirements.
2. Without violating industrial confidentiality, it is necessary to provide clear information about goals and details of the project.
3. Regular, open and honest communication.
4. Flexibility to adapt to biobank conditions and capabilities, including the period required for collecting samples and their associated annotations.
5. Respect amongst partners, considering biobanks as partners and not only as service providers and establishing permanent relationships with common benefits.

Public-private partnerships in biobanking represent the general framework of dialogue where stable or occasional collaborations are established. They are more an attitude than a contract. They form the basis for discussions about agreements looking for win-win situations, and should be established through a global contract of collaboration in case of a stable relationship for a particular scientific goal. Nevertheless, if on this basis a specific action is challenged it is mandatory to formalise it in a well-structured and comprehensive Material Transfer Agreement, in case of a specific project or action [31]. This global contract and, when applicable, Material Transfer Agreement should clearly include and clarify aspects of intellectual property, mutual recognition as equals, and full-cost economical aspects for services rendered.

"WHY" PPP IS MORE IMPORTANT THAN "HOW" WE SHOULD DO IT

In summary, a PPP means more than a specific transfer of samples from a public biobank to an industry-funded group of researchers. It means an environment of discussion and collaboration for the creation of win-win situations.

To consider PPPs in biobanking only in terms of sustainability is an erroneous and incomplete view. They are mainly necessary for a higher goal: social health and welfare, and a better future for specific patients and individuals.

PPP in biobanking should be oriented towards more strategic and relevant goals than a good client-provider relationship. Rather, stable relationships and compromises are the issues that must be dealt with, and they should be entirely in favour of society. The central goal is to provide public service from the public and private sectors as a whole, where mutual trust, transparency and open dialogue are the basic key ingredients.

These key ingredients form the framework for the "how". Academic medicine depends more than ever on public trust. If the public perceive academic medical research institutions, including biobanks, as gaining inappropriately from relations with industry, this will decrease the donors' trust and hence adversely affect the number of donations [32]. As said before, transparency and observing the law are essential ingredients for a correct and fruitful public-private partnership in biobanking.

CONFLICT OF INTEREST

The authors confirm that they have no conflict of interest to declare for this publication.

ACKNOWLEDGEMENT

Spanish National Biobank Network is funded with public funds from the Instituto de Salud Carlos III, under the Health Strategic Actions 2010-2013 (RD09/0076) and 2014-2017 (PT13/0010).

REFERENCES

[1]   Morente MM, Fernández PL, de Alava E. Biobanking: old activity or young discipline? Semin Diagn Pathol 2008; 25(4): 317-22.
        [http://dx.doi.org/10.1053/j.semdp.2008.07.007] [PMID: 19013897]

[2]   Riegman PH, Morente MM, Betsou F, de Blasio P, Geary P. Biobanking for better healthcare. Mol Oncol 2008; 2(3): 213-22.
        [http://dx.doi.org/10.1016/j.molonc.2008.07.004] [PMID: 19383342]

[3]   Zatloukal K, Hainaut P. Human tissue biobanks as instruments for drug discovery and development: impact on personalized medicine. Biomarkers Med 2010; 4(6): 895-903.
        [http://dx.doi.org/10.2217/bmm.10.104] [PMID: 21133710]

[4]   Luijten PR, van Dongen GA, Moonen CT, Storm G, Crommelin DJ. Public-private partnerships in translational medicine: concepts and practical examples. J Control Release 2012; 161(2): 416-21.
        [http://dx.doi.org/10.1016/j.jconrel.2012.03.012] [PMID: 22465390]

[5]   Anderlik M. Commercial biobanks and genetic research: ethical and legal issues. Am J Pharmacogenomics 2003; 3(3): 203-15.
        [http://dx.doi.org/10.2165/00129785-200303030-00006] [PMID: 12814328]

[6]   Stevens AJ, Jensen JJ, Wyller K, Kilgore PC, Chatterjee S, Rohrbaugh ML. The role of public-sector research in the discovery of drugs and vaccines. N Engl J Med 2011; 364(6): 535-41.
        [http://dx.doi.org/10.1056/NEJMsa1008268] [PMID: 21306239]

[7]   Stossel TP. Regulating academic-industrial research relationships solving problems or stifling progress? N Engl J Med 2005; 353(10): 1060-5.
        [http://dx.doi.org/10.1056/NEJMsb051758] [PMID: 16148294]

[8]   Steinbrook R. Financial conflicts of interest and the NIH. N Engl J Med 2004; 350(4): 327-30.
        [http://dx.doi.org/10.1056/NEJMp038247] [PMID: 14736923]

[9]   Clément B, Yuille M, Zaltoukal K, *et al*. Public biobanks: calculation and recovery of costs. Sci Transl Med 2014; 6(261): 261fs45.
[http://dx.doi.org/10.1126/scitranslmed.3010444] [PMID: 25378642]

[10]   Gonzalez-Sanchez MB, Lopez-Valeiras E, Morente MM, Fernández Lago O. Cost model for biobanks. Biopreserv Biobank 2013; 11(5): 272-7.
[http://dx.doi.org/10.1089/bio.2013.0021] [PMID: 24835258]

[11]   Vaught J, Rogers J, Carolin T, Compton C. Biobankonomics: developing a sustainable business model approach for the formation of a human tissue biobank. J Natl Cancer Inst Monogr 2011; 2011(42): 24-31.
[http://dx.doi.org/10.1093/jncimonographs/lgr009] [PMID: 21672892]

[12]   ESFRI (Strategy report on research infrastructures) Roadmap 2010. Luxembourg, Publications Office of the European Union European Union 2011. Available from: http://ec.europa.eu/research/infrastructures/pdf/esfri-strategy_report_and_roadmap.pdf

[13]   Mahan S, Ardlie KG, Krenitsky KF, Walsh G, Clough G. Collaborative design for automated DNA storage that allows for rapid, accurate, large-scale studies. Assay Drug Dev Technol 2004; 2(6): 683-9.
[http://dx.doi.org/10.1089/adt.2004.2.683] [PMID: 15674026]

[14]   Hofman P, Bréchot C, Zatloukal K, Dagher G, Clément B. Public-private relationships in biobanking: a still underestimated key component of open innovation. Virchows Arch 2014; 464(1): 3-9.
[http://dx.doi.org/10.1007/s00428-013-1524-z] [PMID: 24337181]

[15]   LEWIS G. Tissue Collection and the Pharmaceutical Industry: investigating corporate biobanks. In: Tutton R, Corrigan O, Eds. Genetic Databases Socio-ethical issues in the collection and use of DNA. London: Routledge 2004; pp. 181-202.

[16]   Womack C, Gray NM. Banking human tissue for research: vision to reality. Cell Tissue Bank 2009; 10(3): 267-70.
[http://dx.doi.org/10.1007/s10561-008-9104-1] [PMID: 18618293]

[17]   Common minimum technical standards and protocols for biological resource centres dedicated to cancer research, Work Group Report 2. IARC 2007.

[18]   Best Practices for Repositories: Collection, Storage, Retrieval and Distribution of Biological Materials for Research. 3rd ed., Campbell 2011.

[19]   NCI Best Practices for Biospecimen Resources 2014. Available from: http://biospecimens.cancer.gov/bestpractices/2011-NCIBestPractices.pdf

[20]   Biobanks for Europe - A Challenge for Governance. Luxembourg: Publications Office of the European Union 2012. Available from: http://www.coe.int/t/dg3/healthbioethic/Activities/10_Biobanks/biobanks_for_Europe.pdf

[21]   Morente MM, Cereceda L, Luna-Crespo F, Artiga MJ. Managing a biobank network. Biopreserv Biobank 2011; 9(2): 187-90.
[http://dx.doi.org/10.1089/bio.2011.0005] [PMID: 24846266]

[22]   Riegman PH, Dinjens WN, Oomen MH, *et al*. TuBaFrost 1: Uniting local frozen tumour banks into a European network: an overview. Eur J Cancer 2006; 42(16): 2678-83.
[http://dx.doi.org/10.1016/j.ejca.2006.04.031] [PMID: 17027254]

[23]   Vaught J, Kelly A, Hewitt R. A review of international biobanks and networks: success factors and key benchmarks. Biopreserv Biobank 2009; 7(3): 143-50.
[http://dx.doi.org/10.1089/bio.2010.0003] [PMID: 24835880]

[24]   Asslaber M, Zatloukal K. Biobanks: transnational, European and global networks. Brief Funct Genomic Proteomic 2007; (6): 193-201.

[25]   Luscombe NM, Babu MM, Yu H, Snyder M, Teichmann SA, Gerstein M. Genomic analysis of regulatory network dynamics reveals large topological changes. Nature 2004; 431(7006): 308-12.

[http://dx.doi.org/10.1038/nature02782] [PMID: 15372033]

[26]   Hansson MG. For the safety and benefit of current and future patients. Pathobiology 2007; 74(4): 198-205.
         [http://dx.doi.org/10.1159/000104445] [PMID: 17709960]

[27]   Jack AL, Womack C. Why surgical patients do not donate tissue for commercial research: review of records. BMJ 2003; 327(7409): 262.
         [http://dx.doi.org/10.1136/bmj.327.7409.262] [PMID: 12896938]

[28]   Carey N. What do biotech companies want? (Dissertation). Wales Cancer Bank meeting on: "Tissue Banking in the NHS"The advantages for Pathology Departments" 2010. Available from: http://www.walescancerbank.com/tissue-banking-in-the-nhs.htm

[29]   Betsou F, Luzergues A, Carter A, *et al.* Towards Norms for Accreditation of Biobanks for Human Health and Medical Research: Compilation of Existing Guidelines into an ISO Certification / Accreditation Norm-compatible Format. Qual Assur J 2007; 11: 219-92.
         [http://dx.doi.org/10.1002/qaj.425]

[30]   Bevilacqua G, Bosman F, Dassesse T, *et al.* The role of the pathologist in tissue banking: European Consensus Expert Group Report. Virchows Arch 2010; 456(4): 449-54.
         [http://dx.doi.org/10.1007/s00428-010-0887-7] [PMID: 20157825]

[31]   Cervo S, De Paoli P, Mestroni E, *et al.* Drafting biological material transfer agreement: a ready-to-sign model for biobanks and biorepositories. Int J Biol Markers 2016; 31(2): e211-7.
         [http://dx.doi.org/10.5301/jbm.5000190] [PMID: 26868333]

[32]   Angell M. Is academic medicine for sale? N Engl J Med 2000; 342(20): 1516-8.
         [http://dx.doi.org/10.1056/NEJM200005183422009] [PMID: 10816191]

CHAPTER 2

Models of Collaboration and Experiences between Bio-Industry and Academic Biobanks

Rita T. Lawlor* and **Aldo Scarpa**

ARC-Net, Applied Research on Cancer Center, University of Verona, Italy

Abstract: Access to high quality human biological samples and associated medical information is an essential prerequisite to biomedical research and innovation for both academia and industry. In particular, the private industry sector needs access to biospecimens and data to develop innovative products to keep or gain market leadership. Interaction between industry and academia is important from a social and economic stand point. One provides sustainable global economy while the other contributes to the scientific knowledge base. The main challenge in such collaborations is reconciling perceived altruism and open collaboration with intellectual property and profit. In order to establish a fruitful collaboration, the partners need to recognize their differences to produce positive outcomes for both and avoid the potential drawbacks that different cultures can encur when attempting to join forces. As seen in previous chapter, biobanking is indeed a liaison between the public and private realms. Models for partnerships must be characterized by a common vision, shared mutually agreed goals, clear commitment and investment from all partners through formalized collaboration and shared decision-making.This chapter focuses on the elements necessary for successful collaboration between public and private realms and looks at various models of collaborations, from traditional models,that existed before biobanking was recognized as a discipline, to recent models of public-private partnership. These include models directly created for private collaborations with biobanks as well as models of collaboration where biobanks play an integral part. The chapter concludes with suggestions for innovative models of public-private synergy in biobanking for the future.

Keywords: Charitable-trust, Consortia, Data banks, Expert centers, Honest-broker, Intellectual property, National biobank, Networks, Public trust, Research, Safe-harbor, Service, Umbrella initiative, Validation studies.

INTRODUCTION

In a perfect world, a perfect model of collaboration would be one where the tangible and intangible investment of the various partners is recognized and

* **Corresponding Author Rita T. Lawlor**: ARC-Net, Applied Research on Cancer Center, University of Verona, Italy; Tel: 39 045 8127431; Email: rita.lawlor@arc-net.it

Elena Salvaterra and Julie Corfield (Eds.)
All rights reserved-© 2017 Bentham Science Publishers

valued. Translating this principle to biomedical research means that biobanks and public health care systems would have full recognition for the true value of the cost of collecting and annotating the samples, including the entire effort of clinicians, pathologists, nurses, technical personnel that process and collate the information. The university system would have acknowledgement for the education and training they provide to create the minds that invest in these systems, and for their investment in technological platforms and basic research that informs the later processes of translational and applied research.Private industry would have the benefit of the biobanks samples and data and reduced R&D costs through collaboration with academia to develop companion diagnostics and therapies [1]. All of this would feed back into a public benefit to the health care system from which all originates by providing lower costs diagnostic tools and pharmaceuticals. However, this is not a perfect world so no model of collaboration is perfect. From this perspective, we present a series of models of public-private partnership (PPP) in biobanking which include basic traditional forms of collaboration that still function on a smaller scale and more innovative models that attempt to approach this idea of a perfect world and suggest some to fuel those already envisioned.

PPP COLLABORATORS

Models of collaboration intrinsically depend on the type of partners involved in the collaboration itself. So before looking at the possible models for collaboration between public and private realms, it is important to consider the collaborators, understand their point of view, and look at the elements of synergy to evaluate what models work best for certain situations.

Academic Biobank Structures

The academic environment is very heterogeneous. It encompasses undergraduate and graduate education and a diverse faculty with disparate goals and measures of success. The basic scientist has to publish, the clinician is promoted based on doing good clinical work and disseminating that knowledge, and the clinician scientist is trying to expand the translation of science to patients and expand patient care beyond the institution. It is usually either the clinician and/or principal investigator (they may be one and the same) who has contacts with industry. Through collaborations with industry, academia may possibly access increased funding, potentially increase its output through publications and, in some cases, become part of international networks. They are also afforded the opportunity to do research on the advanced end of the research process in the biomedical field to help produce something that is more effective than a costly patent. The relationship that the biobank has with its hospital and academic contributors will affect its involvement in any collaboration. Biobanks that are an integral part of a larger infrastructure such as a research center will have more extensive platforms at its disposal. They will also have the capacity to develop internal research projects and their collaborations will be facilitated by these add on services.

Industry Partner

The bio-industry that requires access to biobanks and biospecimens divides itself into two groups, companion diagnostics and the pharmaceutical industry. It has been easier for the former to collaborate with academia and academic or public hospital biobanks on validation studies for the diagnostic test as the amount and treatment of information required to validate diagnostic tests does not, in general, infringe on the privacy of the patient or healthy individual acting as a control. Pharmaceutical companies,have historically performed the majority of their drug discovery research in house and only collaborated at the stage of clinical trials, The era of industry sustaining completely in-house R&D activities has gone [2, 3]. Industry have realized that they need to change their research models to remain viable. Industry must find ways to outsource these activities and academia has the resources to potentially respond. This has created the possibility for new models of collaboration with academia in order to perform research and with biobanks as the underlying research infrastructure and the provider of samples and data.

Small and Medium Enterprises

(SMEs) have the most to gain by collaborating with academia. As they have limited research resources, collaborating with academia affords them greater research capabilities and platforms with which to execute important validation studies. SMEs have less administrative structure, which can be a double edge sword. While it means they can be more flexible, it also means that less structure within the private organization combined with the un-structured academic research approach can be detrimental to achieving a result. It does however create a more open environment when discussing issues of intellectual property. SMEs fit more comfortably into the mission of academia as they are seen as one step beyond a university spin-off. Collaboration with SMEs, if carried out within the university are then considered part of the invaluable education and progression the university must provide for its researchers [4].

Government & Public

The general public is the partner that should gain the most from any partnership. The end result of any efficient research cycle is the provision of more cost-efficient and targeted treatment and thus an improvement in health care services.

ELEMENTS TO BE ADDRESSED IN MODELS OF COLLABORATION

Partnerships are successful when all participants benefit. Academia is more involved in the earlier phases of research, particularly basic research, and there are no particular timelines involved in this. In comparison Industry works at the latter end of the process in the clinical and applied research portions where time is of the essence and it is part of the bottom line to get the technology or product to market. The two meet somewhere in the middle in translational research where both are taking an idea from basic research and attempting to translate it to a project that can produce an application (Fig. **1**).

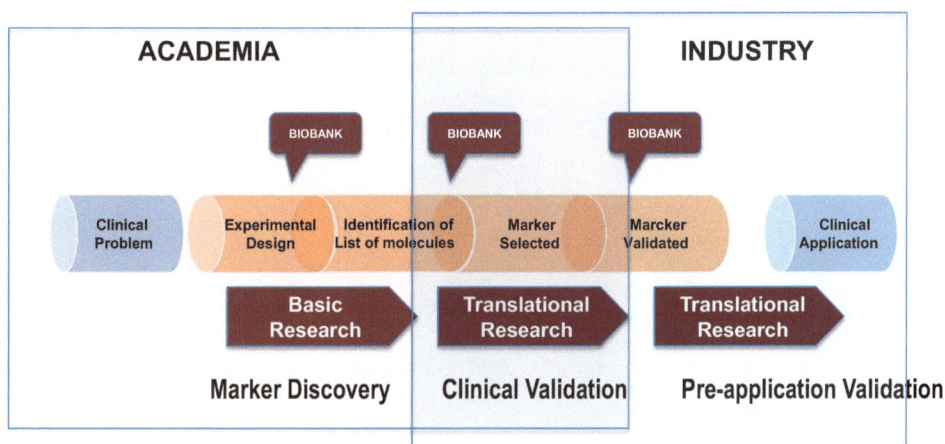

Fig. (1). The process form discovery to application and the parts the collaborators play in the process.

Numerous elements affect the success of public private collaborations, many of which are cultural (Table **1**). It is important that all partners in public-private collaborations acknowledge that their backgrounds, make-up and objectives are different. There are also the historic questions of fairness to the biobank donating public/ biobank contributing medical personnel and facilitating access to materials for research and stimulating innovation. Numerous conferences have addressed these issues in recent years (Hands on Biobanking Uppsala 2012, European, Middle Eastern and Africa Society for Biopreservation and Biobanking 2013, Hands on Biobanking, Helsinki 2014) but it is important that they are clearly elocuted in any collaboration agreement to avoid misunderstandings and eventual collapse of collaborations (1).

Different Goals

The main goal of the academic institution is education and research and its success is evaluated in research funding and publications. Meanwhile, the goal of bio-industry is to produce technologies and products and their success is measured in terms of profit generated. It is important that the specific objective of collaborations respond to these different foundation goals. These may be potentially at odds, as academia wants to publish results as soon as possible whereas the private partner wants to have exclusive access to these to maintain market advantage. As such, it is important that the timing of release of results is discussed to ensure that everyone's needs are satisfied. For the biobank, this will be more or less important, depending on its level of participation and often the biobank will be stuck in the middle, requiring both the recognition through the publication but also needing to demonstrate its capacity to provide samples for valid and reproducible research (2-4).

Table 1. Examples of epialleles in plants (modified from Richards, 2006; Pilu, 2015).

ACADEMIA	INDUSTRY
Early phases in drug discovery	Later phases in drug application
Knowledge, publications, grants, new research	Information, products, sales, profit
Open access to results	Exclusive access to results
Need to publish results as soon as possible	Need to put moratorium on results to translate results into products
Long term research projects	Short term research projects
Open research questions leading to novel discoveries	Market driven research linked to "proprietary" compounds / technology
Tightening of research funding puts strain on academic research	Falling profits have created the necessity for outsourcing of R&D
"Give me the money and I will tell you when I have something"	"Give me the results and I will evaluate the market potential value"

Different Concepts of Time

Public and private entities work to different time lines. While the private sector are used to working to project plans and deadlines, the concept of time in the academic research world is more flexible notion. As such any collaboration, particularly a one-to-one collaboration, must have clear definitions and timelines included with monitoring systems to review, take note and adjust accordingly.

IP and other Returns

Industry is genetically equipped to monitor return on investment. A private company needs to provide product, in the form of services, technology or reagents, to its sales force in order to respond to its through revenue and profit. It is always aware of its return in any agreement and it is less concerned with IP, rather its concerns in this regard are with exclusive access and license. Academia too has interests to protect such as the interests of the clinicians and scientists involved in any collaboration. Academia is more concerned with IP and to a lesser extent patents as this is the academic way to protect the interests of collaborating scientists and basic research results. Therefore, with the exception of clinical trials that have very specific objectives, collaboration agreements usually include conditions regarding IP and patents. Now, in the era of open access, these issues are becoming less important for those wishing to publish (5, 6). Biobanks live in a world where it can often be difficult to understand where compensation ends and profit begins. Although samples are considered the basic fuel of research, they are not considered part of the actual research effort, thus there is no full acknowledgement in the resulting product or publication. Usually, biobanks also have no property rights to the samples or data and therefore, no intellectual property, background or otherwise, can be assigned. Even if IP could be assigned to primary samples, it would be lost once the sample is manipulated in any way. This places the biobank in difficult position when negotiating intellectual property in the resulting research. Some models of collaboration have tried to change the approach to this [11, 12].

Different Concepts of Collaborations and Contracts

Not only the different languages of public and private sectors,but also their underlying cultures enter into the picture [13, 14]. For academia, collaborations can be open-ended verbal agreements and often the competitive spirit of academia only tends towards the development of contracts for protectionism in the form of patents and names on publications. Contracts, on the other hand, are rigid dark formalities of administration that have little to do with science and seem to be more allied to the world of profit. It is easy to overlook that biobanks have been the first to move into this arena implementing supporting contracts for its exchange activities in the form of materials transfer agreements (MTAs).All collaborations should be underwritten by a document that clearly defines the objectives and expected outcome of the partnership regardless of the model eventually employed and explicates timeframe, materials and methods (as would any scientific project), investment and cost, who is contributing what to the project and who receives what. The latter will include actual payment, up front or periodic, resulting ownership and share in the result be it data, technology, publications or a patentable result. In this case, who has the right, on us or obligation of submitting the patent should be clearly outlined. It is also important to remember that contracts, particularly for long-term agreements, serve to protect the investment in the research as personnel may change over time, especially within the industry and the collaboration may lose its champion. So, while a contract may seem a cold and non-collaborative act at the onset, a contract protects everyone [15, 16].

Conflict of Interest

This is an interesting issue that most affects the public and academic sector in a PPP collaboration where the public interest may conflict with the private interest. Conflict of interest is important as it may potentially undermine impartially of individuals or institutions regarding a specific collaboration. It is, of course not restricted to this one issue nor does it exclude industry. The words "Bad Pharma" are synonymous with pharmaceutical companies who by simulation or dissimulation, either exaggerated results, pushed a certain study or failed to disclose research information regarding side-effects or toxicity. In the arena of academic/public biobanking that deals with the public samples and data usually collected by academic and hospital biobanks, this is the area that most concerns the potential benefits of public private partnerships.

Arguably, it could be considered an issue of self-interest. Where an individual or institution has more than one direct or indirect affiliation, there is the potential for conflict. Such an example is a clinician involved in the care of patients who wants better ways to diagnose patients and better therapies to treat them and therefore becomes involved in research with a company to contribute to the development of diagnostic tools and therapies. Any potential bias that may be introduced into the research regardless of financial reward highlights the conflict that may arise from the desire to help his patients and produce a successful product.

Once personal interests are declared and products are evaluated on merits as the public health care system demands there should be no conflict. One solution is to ensure that scientists who develop novel treatments should not test these treatments on humans. If the biobank acts as the independent collaborator with industry providing the samples and data that the clinician might have provided in the past, the potential for bias and conflict may be alleviated. These issues of perception are often those that most hinder collaboration between public and private [17].

Public Trust

The public has always had mixed feelings regarding the private industry getting access to their samples or data, in part from feelings of mistrust, in part because they feel industry is profiting from them [18, 19]. The exception to this has been clinical trials where the collaboration is more immediate and therefore the public or patient better perceives a quid pro quo and the potential advantage of collaboration. The donor receives reimbursement and the patient, in direct need has access to potentially life saving experimental therapies. This mistrust has increased now that we have moved into the era of research because of the perceived increase in risk for the public. As such, the public already has mixed feelings about genetic research and even more so about whom they trust to have access to their genetic data [20 - 22].

The Wellcome Trust Monitor Wave 2 [23] endeavoured in 2013 to track the views on science, biomedical research and science education. It showed that levels of trust for medical practitioners and scientists working in universities was the same, closely followed by medical research charities at 60%. Interestingly scientists working for government only barely rated higher than scientists working in the private industry and both rated better than government departments and ministers. In the 4 years from 2009 to 2012, trust in doctors has gone down slightly by 5% while trust in university scientists has gone up by 5%. More noteworthy is the fact that, trust in scientists working in industry and government has gone up by 6% so while still way behind on the trust scale perhaps there is hope [23].

A study by Critchley and Nicol [24] suggests that the type of organization, private entity *versus* university, has a greater impact on public trust than the funding source, private *versus* public funding, although the source of funding does assert a certain influence on public trust. While the study did not specifically concern biobanking research, it does suggest that public biobanks, which receive private funding, would better maintain public trust than those that are completely privately owned or funded. This is important as it affects the ability to recruit and retain participants.

Recruitment of Patients

The issue of trust and the perception of profit over benefit [19] will affect both primary recruitment and retention. When private funding is introduced to a pre-existing publicly funded biobank, a concern for the biobank will be retaining participants who were originally recruited on the premises that the biobank was for 'public good' [25]. In this case, issues related to consent, participant retention and withdrawal of biological material and associated data will be particularly important. This contrasts with a biobank that is a public-private partnership from its inception. In this scenario, recruitment of participants and related consent with regard to provision of samples to commercial entities will have been included.

Privacy Issues, Data Sharing and Requirements for Additional Oversight

While these issues are relevant for any biobank, even one that navigates only academic waters, it is an even greater issue when considering a biobank that collaborates with industry, in whatever form. Once again, this feeds from the ideas of public trust and whether the biobank, when applying for ethical approval and creating its informed consent, requested the ability to provide samples or data to a profit based enterprise [18] and thus function in a more ample arena without having to return to the individual for specific consent [26].

Incidental Findings

The handling of incidental findings (IFs) has emerged as one of the most contentious issues within the area of biobanking [27]. This issue may be complicated by the involvement of industry as the user, and therefore the one discovering these incidental findings, will be the industrial partner there may be no provisions to return them to the biobank. To facilitate collaboration with industry, the biobank may have anonymized samples before giving them to the industrial partner and can no longer re-associate the information. These elements should be evaluated carefully when selecting the appropriate model of collaboration.

Issues of Quality

Quality is always the driving force between any potential collaboration. It is directly tied to expectations and sometimes these expectations are considered as given and thus are not described in precise terms. This can result in the failure in the collaboration for failing to meet expectations. It is, thus, vital that all quality parameters that describe elements of the collaboration are specified. The corollary of this is that a biobank that functions with precise parameters of quality has more added value and will function better in a collaboration with industry [28].

The Shift to Data

The intrinsic value of a human sample lies in the information that can be extracted from it using various methods and technologies. This value increases when this intrinsic data can be associated with other information concerning the origin of the sample. Human biological samples are a finite key resource but data cannot be consumed. Furthermore, access to data is much easier than to samples, information can be more easily shared and with lower costs. Data can be made accessible to the broad global scientific community who can create additional and diverse value whereas biological samples can only be provided to a limited group of scientists, and this in turn limits the value-add that can be produced [29]. The future of clinical biobanking will increasingly shift to the provision of high quality data derived from biological samples, rather than provision of the physical biological samples. Cutting edge research as well as future innovations in the life science industry will strongly depend on transnational access to high quality human biological data derived from samples, and to the associated medical information, all of which must be accessible to both academia and industry in an efficient and secure manner. The biobank can thus move from being a sample provider to being a knowledge provider. In fact, many research projects and international collaborations [30] make data freely available under the guard of a data access committee. The concept of making data freely available is not contrary to the potential to generate income. Some of the largest companies today are internet-based companies who make information freely available.

BASIC MODELS OF COLLABORATION

The first set of models presented is based on traditional models of collaboration that have been in place for many years, sometimes in an informal manner. These collaborations are the basis of direct collaborations and are especially functional in collaborations that regard small studies.

Service Based Collaboration

The service based collaboration model typically regards short term, urgent project requirements. The collaboration is based purely on the ability of the biobank to provide the samples, minimum data set and basic services required by the bio-industry company [31]. These services may be activities such as extraction of nucleic acids from tissue or blood.

Service-based collaborations are usually one-to-one agreements that for the most part, mirror the old models of collaboration with regard to the supply of biological materials by public entities to commercial enterprises. They can also expand to one-to-many models where many institutions are providing these samples or services to a single commercial partner. Clinical trials could potentially fall into this type of collaboration.

Advantages

In this model, the term "collaboration" is perhaps incorrect as this model provides a very one directional restrictive environment where the service provider has little or no involvement in the project for which his services are required. The elements indicated previously come less into play. The agreement should be straightforward regarding the services offered but it should be very explicit on timeframe and deadline. As a fee for service agreement, this can be an easy way for the biobank to create an initial rapport with the commercial company and a way to procure some funds for the maintenance and continuation of the biobank. If the biobank has functioned in a patient care and diagnostic environment, it will understand the concept of deadlines and time to response and will not have difficulty in providing the services within the agreed time frame. With this model, there are no lengthy negotiations about intellectual property. The associated data required with the samples can be quite limited, and as long as the samples and data are being provided within the scope of the acquired consents and approvals there is no issue of privacy and data protection [32].

Limitations

In this restricted collaboration model, there is usually little return for the biobank other than financial remuneration for samples in the form of cost recovery and for services. Mention in any resulting publication should the project produce interesting results [3]. This would only happen if the contract indicates this as a requirement either as part of the agreement or as part of the MTA (materials transfer agreement) required before transfer or use of samples for the project. The industry partner benefits from using the name of the biobank in any resulting publication only where the biobank or its scientific personnel carried added value, perhaps due to the biobank's reputation for quality. Resulting data are unlikely to be shared with the biobank and as such there is no added value either for the biobank or for future research [33]. This is unfortunate as it limits the added value of the sample, the availability of the analytical data and the reduction in repeated analyses always assuming that the quality of the analytical research data produced is technologically adequate and compatible with future use.

Research Collaboration Agreement

The research collaboration model can either be a framework agreement under which specific projects are added as, and when, the collaboration progresses or it can regard a specific project and therefore can also be considered the project model. Once again, this model can either be structured as a one-to-one collaboration or one-to-many collaboration although this leads us towards a network structure, which will be discussed later.

The research collaboration model functions best when the biobank is part of a larger context and has additional resources and facilities to bring to the table. This is usually the case when the biobank is part of a larger research infrastructure upon which it can rely to provide the additional research knowledge and execute the necessary study on samples. University hospitals allied to Research Centers are an excellent example of this, where the biobank collection is an integral part of the specific research project design. In this case, the agreement between the private partner and academia is project based financing or considered as commissioning a project [34]. This is usually unrestricted research funding and based on the relationship with the principal investigator.

As with the previous model, these collaborations are very one directional event, where the university carries out all of the research and simply provides results to the commissioning company. In this scenario, there is little research collaboration but both parties'goals are met. The university receives financing for its project and the company gets information that will be useful to its broader strategy. Projects designed in this manner are a good way to initiate a relationship and to test the waters before moving onto more active bi-directional collaborations where lesser autonomy on the part of the university may cause concerns regarding time-lines and deadlines.

Biomarker development and clinical biomarker validation projects lend themselves successfully to this kind of collaboration where pharmaceutical companies request that the university investigates molecular anomalies on a set of samples that respond to particular criteria from its biobank collection or to investigate molecular pathways as potential targets for targeted therapies [35].

Advantages

The biobank becomes a partner in the biomarker research team and is directly involved in the development of the project. In this way, costs/ investment are distributed among the partners, as are the benefits. The biobank's samples and data could be considered as background IP and part of its investment in the project. Depending on the activities required by the project, the biobank could provide additional services for some remuneration, similar to the service based model but adjusted for its role in the project. The biobank can then benefit based on its investment from any produced intellectual property that results from the research.

Limitations

Contracts for such collaborations require IP clauses although in the example of unrestricted grants, IP would belong to the university but the company would have first refusal on an exclusive license to use the IP. In collaborations such as these, the university has complete freedom to organize and carry out the research. However, when the collaboration is being financed by a single entity, payment is usually tied to short-term periodic milestones (interim results / reports) in order to ensure that the project time line is respected. This can be a little daunting for academia to have to respond to such constrictions on time.

Moving to a One to Many Situation

Both the service and the research collaboration models function well in a one-to - one structure. However, the further along the research process the larger the sample size and so for larger scale validation studies, these models have greater power in a networked structure although they require more interaction and greater governance between the collaborators [36, 37].

Onconetwork Consortium

This is a specific example of research collaboration where the company went to its customer base to create a consortium for a validation study (Fig. **2**). Thermo Fisher Scientific set up a consortium of translational cancer research institutes that not only had Life technologies next generation sequencing facilities in a research context but also had access to biobanked cancer samples and associated data regarding the molecular diagnosis of the patient donors. The idea behind the "community panel" was to create NGS panels using expertise from medical and scientific community to characterize a range of diseases that would be useful in research and clinical settings.

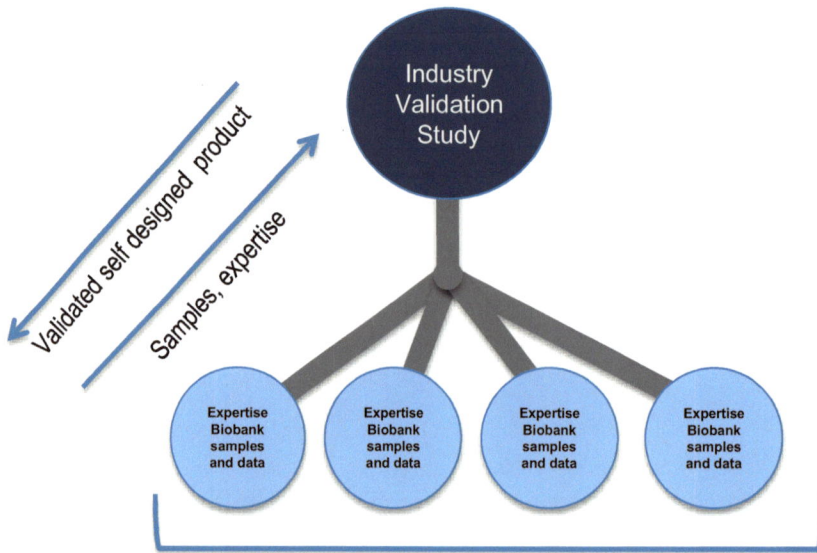

Fig. (2). The structure of a validation study consortium.

The first project of the Onconetwork consortium [38] pertained to the development of a community panel for lung and colon cancer. A panel was designed and tested by seven different laboratories in their own clinical settings. Samples used in the project came from the collaborating institutions. All samples were anonymized and as the study was considered a service improvement, it did not require specific research ethics committee approval as stated in the EU Clinical Trials Directive (2001/20/EC). The first phase aimed at confirming the accuracy and precision of the panel. Consortia labs tested control samples in an inter-laboratory 'ring-trial'. The second phase comprised a ring-trial in which laboratories provided samples from their biobank to be tested by a second consortium laboratory. The third phase of the validation study was to confirm the panel on typically small diagnostic samples.

Data Access is Easier in Validation Studies

This example highlights the ease of collaborating with bio-tech companies requiring access to samples for validation purposes only, as less patient associated data is required facilitating the data access process. In this example, only pathology diagnosis and mutations routinely identified in molecular diagnostic tests, were required.

Validation Studies Rarely Have Intellectual Property Issues

This example of validation studies is easier than many not only for the ease of access of samples due to the need for only minimal data but also due to the fact that intellectual property is not an issue as the base technology has already been developed by the bio-tech company and therefore is not an element of the collaboration.

Academia Advantage

While the collaboration and services provided do extend slightly beyond the remit of a biobank of today, it is certainly in the realms of biobanking activities where the possibility to molecularly characterize the individual provides a more valuable sample to potential users. The Onconetwork collaboration also provided biobank and clinical researchers with the opportunity to provide input and contribute to the panel design. This has been the subject of abstracts and publications [39] and as such provided the academic partner and therefore the biobank with its most valuable payment in impact factor points.

Industry Advantage

The idea behind the "community panel" is that it avails of the expertise of scientific leaders and the NGS community to create NGS panels to characterize a range of diseases.

Limitations

Potential conflict of interest is the greatest element to be addressed in validation study collaborations, although the issue can be amortized by collaborating in a networked structure. Furthermore, should the collaborating centers not gain financially from the collaboration, the potential conflict is eliminated. Of course, in this case, the biobank then needs a different mechanism to recover its costs which can be difficult as the validation itself takes precedence as reflected in resulting publications and the contribution of the samples is often lost. This is an age-old problem that persists to this day and often regardless of model or industry participation [40].

Need For Modification of Models Of Collaboration

This collaboration with industry goes beyond a simple provision of samples. It includes the provision of intellectual expertise and technological infrastructure that extends from expertise in extracting nucleic acids from difficult samples and providing extensive quality control to next generation sequencing infrastructure and know-how that as yet may not currently be considered as part of standard biobanking facilities. It speaks to the fact that biobanks can increase the services they provide or ally themselves with technological experts to provide an interesting and sustainable package.

BIOBANK SPECIFIC MODELS OF COLLABORATION

The previous set of models presented collaborations in terms of not only biobank collections but also had the biobank embedded with additional services and research. The next set of models is specific to biobanks and presents the models possible for public and private entities to collaborate to manage biobank collections and biobank specific services.

Broker Model

The example presented above is an interesting novel model where the single bio-industry company creates its direct specific network. Traditionally, a broker is an interface company that acts on behalf of the bio-industry partner to put together or access samples and data to fit the requirements of the study (Fig. **3**) [41].

One Size Fits Alls

A private broker model is an intermediary for all partners and requirements. The broker can just as easily source samples from its network of academic or hospital biobanks or from the collections in the possession of pharmaceutical companies. The broker has the ability to put together any size or type of partner as long as the samples meet the requirements and can be put together based on criteria and quality.

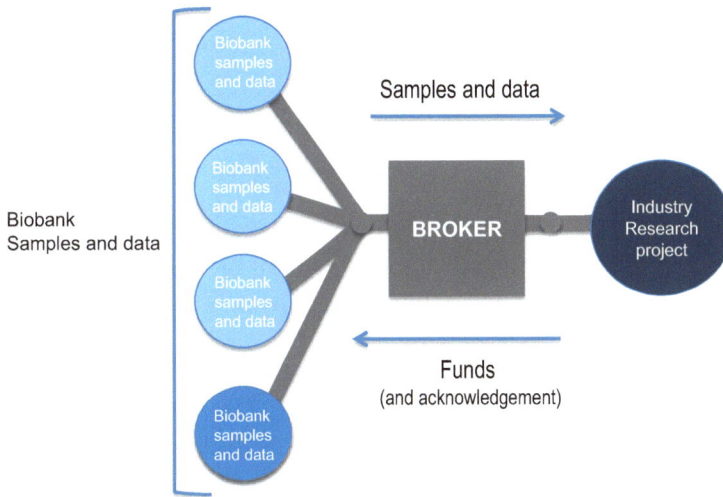

Fig. (3). The broker model that acquires samples and data from various biobanks for individual or multiple industry research programs.

The Honest Broker

Placing an intermediary between the biobank or hospital collection and the industry partner ensures that samples are coded in a similar manner and increase the sample anonymization process. This is a definite advantage as the issue of anonymization and privacy can tend be handled in a less standardized and protected manner for biobanks that work within a diagnostic environment and at times a clear line is not drawn.

Limitations in Accessing Standard Data

An issue that these brokers have in trying to put together samples from different collections is the difficulty in harmonizing sample quality. The situation is exacerbated when it comes to accessing and harmonizing the associated and follow-up data regarding the patient from which the sample was retrieved [42].

National Broker Model

This is a recent development in biobanking. A biobank or specific collection that was part of large research project or population study can be taken over by a private partner who is the interface for this specific collection. They can then set the premise to become a national broker and acquire other collections to make them available for wider studies, having the competence and know-how to provide adequate governance for access to these samples and data. One example of this is presented below and indicates how this model can provide correct governance and facilitated access for collaboration between public and private enterprises.

Lifandis

HUNT Biosciences AS was created to provide service offerings based on data and biologic materials from the renowned cohort samples of the Nord-Trøndelag Health Study (HUNT) with more than 130,000 individuals contributing to the comprehensive population-based databank and biological material biobank. It changed its name to Lifandis to extend the scope of service offerings by acquiring other collections. Lifandis is a commercial interface between industry and the Nord-Trøndelag Health Study (HUNT) and provides commercial access to this collection without compromising the trust of the donor population. It is owned by the Norwegian University of Science and Technology, the Central Norway Health Authority and the Nord-Trøndelag County [43].

The information generated in the HUNT studies is treated according to the guidelines of the Data Inspectorate. The Data Inspectorate of Norway and the Central Norway Regional Committee for Medical and Health Research Ethics in Norway (REK) have approved the HUNT samples for genetic studies. If data from other (national) health registries shall be accessed and merged with HUNT data, the approval from The Directorate for Health and Social Affairs is required.

Importantly, the Central Norwegian Health Research Ethics (REK) recently decided that biological material and data generated in the HUNT surveys can be used in projects with commercial partners based on the existing informed consent. Projects using biological material and data from the HUNT studies have to be approved by the Regional Committee for Medical and Health Research Ethics (REK). Lifandis has been able to collaborate in varying projects due to its set-up. These have ranged from a validation study on a biomarker discovery for a proteomics company to a preventive intervention study.

Safe Harbour

As has been mentioned, the general public continues to have a negative attitude towards commercialization and industry collaboration with biobanks concerning access to samples and data. Norway is no different in this respect, however the model of Lifandis enables collaboration with Industry in a manner that is accepted by the Norwegian public. This is no doubt due to the idea of a non-profit interface between the two that acts in the interest of the donors by setting up committees to evaluate each request and the governance structure that evaluates access.

Win-Win

Lifandis serves as an access platform between the biobank and the Private sector and can use its knowledge of both sectors to ensure that all requirements of both sides are met. While a standard MTA is available, a legally binding contract, it is customized to address each individual agreement. Lifandis also handles project management, which is another of the areas where the two worlds do not speak the same language and this benefits both parties. One very big advantage is that the public entity in this case, the University, gets economic funding. Lifandis' profits go to the university. Furthermore the researchers that were involved in the biobank collection are included in the research project as authors of any eventual manuscripts that support the individual's academic career. This inception of the broker model, with its ability to provide other services moves its concept towards a more innovative model that will be discussed later.

Limitations

While the samples and data remain the "property" of HUNT, the results of the individual projects become the property of the commercial partner in the project. As there is no return of data to the biobank, this limits what is available to future requesters of the biobank.

Public – Private National/Population Biobank Model

This model requires that the collaboration be envisaged, usually before the creation of the biobank. There are a number of advantages of this model over the public biobank or those mainly embedded in larger public infrastructures. They have a clearer idea of their investment, have a strategy for sustainability and a business plan from the outset. The private investment requires no modification to the original governance structure, as it is tailor made to its investment description. This means there are no concerns about public trust and re-consenting as the donors are aware from the start about the investment. In this model and the examples below most of the private investment came from chartable foundations and not-for-profit organizations but this was not the deciding factor in success or failure.

Danish National Biobank Example

The Danish National Biobank [44] is a collaboration between the public and private sectors in Denmark. It is financed largely by the Novo Nordisk Foundation [45], with contributions from the Lundbeck Foundation and the Danish Government Programme for Research Infrastructure. The biobank is a state-of -the-art Biobank with the most advanced technology to perform specific assays on samples. The biobank is also connected to national registries and has an open access policy. The ability to collate data and samples from various registries provides immense opportunities for epidemiological studies. It does however open questions about data protection and ethics and the opt-out policy of the country with regard to being part of national medical registries that contain medical histories and genetic code.

Power in Numbers

There are a number such models of national biobank particularly in the Nordic European countries such as Estonia (Estonia Genome Foundation) and Norway (Biobank Norway, Lifandis) who have also joined forces under a network, the Nordic Biobank Network [46] and are part of the larger European biobanking research infrastructure (BBMRI-ERIC). This shows value of a single united front with regard to a particular biobanking activity to provide an integrated resource whose potential is an exponential aggregate of the individual elements.

A Cautionary Tale

The first attempt at this type of model occurred in Iceland with the launch of DeCode Genetics. The intention was to perform research on genes and DNA but the structure of the collaboration raised many questions. In brief, the Icelandic Government agreed to give DeCode Genetics, a commercial company, access to health records to create a database and to ensure co-operation of the entire population. The intention was no doubt altruistic but as it was investigating inheritable genetics alterations, it ran into a legal battle due to the potential to infringe on the privacy of even non-participants. deCODE Genetics went into bankruptcy, emerged under Saga Investments and was then purchased in 2012 by Amgen [47] and the genetics database became NextCODE Health. Although the database belonged to the National Health System, deCODE has access to the database. It could deny access to others if it were against their financial interests yet it could make data available to other commercial companies for a price. This has caused two opposing concerns, the first was the public feeling that they have been exploited by a commercial entity. On the other hand there is the problem that now genetic anomalies have been identified but there is no means to make this available for the benefit of public health [48]. This begs the question "is this the right thing for the wrong reason, the wrong thing for the right reason, or somewhere in between?"

Charitable Trust and Beyond

The charitable Trust model [49] moves to the consideration of ethics in terms of the collective and not focused on the individual. For such a consideration to function, the biobank must be considered as a common resource and access to the resource is handled through institutional representative governance. This model also goes towards addressing issues of open access and potential misuse of data. As a not-for-profit organization, it stands in the middle of the public-private spectrum and evokes a larger community identity of the honest broker.

The UK Biobank Example

UK Biobank [50] was established by the Wellcome Trust medical charity [51], the Medical Research Council [52], Department of Health [53], Scottish Government [54] and the Northwest Regional Development Agency. It has also had funding from the Welsh Assembly Government, British Heart Foundation and Diabetes UK. UK Biobank is hosted by the University of Manchester and supported by the National Health Service (NHS). UK Biobank is a registered not-for-profit charity in its own right, with the aim of improving the prevention, diagnosis and treatment of a wide range of serious and life-threatening illnesses. It is an open access resource open to bona fide scientists, undertaking health-related research that is in the public good. Approved scientists from academia, government, charity and commercial companies can request access to the biobank. UK Biobank requests return of results deemed of interest to the global research community and acknowledgement that "this research has been conducted using the UK Biobank Resource [55].

Public Trust

The advantage of this model is that the biobank is the main focus of the collaboration on two levels. The main goal of the collaboration is to create a biobank and set up not only the physical infrastructure to support it but also the governance structure to administer to it. The involvement of national government bodies and not-for-profit foundations as its founding members allies all concerns of public trust regarding public and private access and intervention. The Board of Directors has a Medical Research Council member and a Department of Health member as indirect representation for the public. While the UK Biobank asserts ownership of the samples and data, the creation of an Ethics and Governance Framework and the introduction of public consultations [56] have moved this notion towards a form of soft public ownership, facilitating benefit sharing to both academia and industry and protecting the rights of the public and the research community at large [57].

NEW MODELS OF COLLABORATION

The era of genomic sequencing and personalized medicine has created the need to provide next generation diagnostics. They have also provided the opportunity for the use of biomarkers and targeted therapies. These opportunities have created an increased need for pharmaceutical companies, biotechnology companies, academia and public to find new ways to collaborate to find more answers to the personalized medicine question of which biobanks have become a recognized element. Below are two new models of PPP collaboration that move to the greater need for coordination and harmonization on a larger scale to be able to address the bigger questions.

Expert Center Model

The concept of the expert center is a model of biobanking that enables public private cooperation by incorporating elements from the other models to address the issues of concern with collaborations between public and private. As seen previously, the ability to provide added value for the biobank in the form of additional services places the biobank in a better situation to collaborate.

The concept of a neutral interface is important as it addresses the primary issue of public trust by providing the safe harbor for collaboration while combining the perspectives of the various stakeholders, the biobank participants' requirements for privacy with industries' requirement for samples. The ability to de-humanize the samples by performing molecular characterization and expanding the sample into a data representation of its components under different analytical assays provides the privacy, anonymization, service and reporting all in one (Fig. **4**).

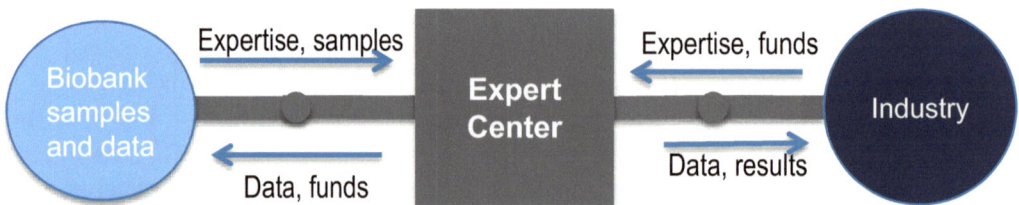

Fig. (4). The expert center is the "analytical broker" that acts as the intermediary transforming samples and associated information into analytical data for industry applications.

Expert centers are an extension of the public private collaboration of old where the public institution, which had access to the interesting set of biological specimens and the technological capabilities to carry out activities to answer research questions would enter a project based collaboration agreement as described earlier in the chapter.

The expert center model is an extension of this as it also introduces a degree of separation between the biobank and the industry, similar to the model of honest broker, but has the added advantage of dealing only with analyzed data. The public-private, ideally not-for-profit expert center would be the safe harbor, and would perform the molecular analyses on the selected samples for the requested and approved study whose results would be supplied. In this way, donors' material would not move out of the biobanking infrastructure, and data would be stored for re-use in other studies [58].

This feeds into the trend of considering everything in terms of data and this facilitates exchange between various partners and indeed across country borders where exchange of samples might have been prohibitive. The compound interest of increasing amounts of qualified analytic data available for association with the biological samples potentially creates a true benefit sharing opportunity for both academia and industry.

An important element of expert centers goes to addressing concerns of privacy and protection. The intention of this separation between biobank and techno-logical platform is to ensure that the detailed biological samples and all associated clinical, pathological and pre-analytical sample data remains in the domain of the collecting biobank and its contributing clinicians, pathologists and scientists. This leaves all the concerns of privacy and protection in the hands of those who deal directly with the donor.

BBMRI Expert Centres

The European Biobanking and Biomolecular Resources Research Infrastructure (BBMRI) was created with European funding to improve the accessibility and interoperability of biological samples from different sub-populations of Europe. The infrastructure builds on existing sample collections and biobanking technologies and, integrates these biobanks into a pan-European distributed hub-and-spoke structured network, embedded into national scientific, ethical, legal and societal frameworks. Interoperability is achieved by implementation of common standards and access rules, which consider the heterogeneity of pertinent national legislation and ethical principles. The BBMRI-ERIC example is one that comp-rises elements of different models of collaboration with industry. The biobanks function as a network with an integrated catalogue to present bio-specimen availability to potential collaborative requests. Here however, the focus is on BBMRI developed concept of expert centers that are also part of their network system and provide the technologically functional interface between the biobank facility and the industrial partner. BBMRI Expert Centers are intended to function as a focal point of contact between the public and the private sector. The set-up of BBMRI Expert Centers will be decided on the level of the member countries. Pilot studies are already ongoing and it is envisaged that complete implementation should be co-financed from the public and private sectors, and by using funding instruments provided by the European Investment Bank [59].

An Expansion of Other Models

Just as the expert center can be seen as a broker that manipulates the sample by turning it into analytical data, similarly brokers who provide technological services can be considered expert centers. A case in point is the Lifandis example presented earlier [43], which can also be considered an expert center within the BBMRI-ERIC model. In truth, it is a mixture of models. In this scenario, the private partner acts as an intermediary between the public biobank and all potential industry collaborations but it is also the expert center as it provides analytical services to turn samples into pure data. It is a double chinese wall, it is first the wall between the biobank and bio-industry but it is also the wall that is the expert center providing sample " data translation" services. The advantage of this scenario is that the biobank can remain in the public realm while the "broker" can move towards negotiating with the commercial world. This permits the regulation of data and results between biobank and commercial world. It also provides the ability to qualify data based on the technology and methods used.

A Specific Networked Example Of A BBMRI Expert Center

The EXpert Center in METabolomics (EXCEMET) [60] is a not-for –profit public-private partnership based on a consortium agreement between academia and industry. Its goal is to further develop technologies and standardize procedures for broad application of metabolomics in research and diagnostics. It is a distributed expert center and therefore created as a network of facilities that together form an expert center. Its founding partners are universities and limited companies working in different areas of metanomics and environmental health. The expert center combines all essential analytical and informatics/computational expertise in the field with the main objective to strengthen the relationships between the metabolomics community. EXCEMET complements the activities of the biobanks [61], extending access from high quality samples to advanced biomolecular analyses and the dissemination of curated knowledge from those analyses in open-access, long-term maintained databases. Technical developments focus on precompetitive issues, such as decreasing minimal sample volume, improvement of sample stabilization and assay sensitivity, reduction of experiment time, data analysis and reduction of costs. EXCEMET will provide guidance to biobanks on sample management for metabolomics.

Advantages and Limitations

This is a distributed expert center model uniting centers in different countries where the exchange is through data exchange. It shows the potential of expert centers at their full capacity regarding exchange of only information across borders without the concerns of sharing samples. It is a move into the new era. However, as the example regards metabolomics studies, which are involved with data regarding chemical processes, it does not touch on the sensitive area of genetic data and so avoids the concerns related to this. It is, as such, a safe test bed for this new model functioning in the extended network structure. As seen in earlier models, the potential of all collaboration models is enhanced when biobanks are part of a network that can increase the interest for industry to access larger sets of samples organized in a multi center network and incorporate additional expertise and capabilities. Here too, the BBMRI-ERIC infrastructure is a networked infrastructure and indeed the expert centre model functions in a networked configuration (Fig. **5**) at two levels, the first among centers and the second, as in the EXCEMET example, to create a single expert center from a consortium of centers contributing different expertise.

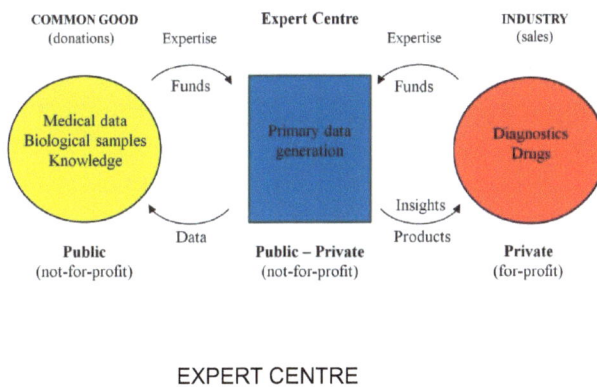

EXPERT CENTRE

Fig. (5). The BBMRI Expert Centre as the key actor providing a trusted, operational middle ground between the public and private sectors copied from http://www.bbmri-lpc.org/ExpertCentres.

But what about a network of networks or a network of projects? This brings us to the way forward in terms of public, private partnerships.

UMBRELLA INITIATIVES

Umbrella Initiatives are public private initiatives that are created based on a specific research theme. They are considered umbrella initiatives because they are created to support collaborative research projects and networks of public and private entities (Fig. **6**). They provide an environment for research and innovation and set out the governance, financing and structure under which these specific projects and networks operate. These initiatives are the essence of precompetitive collaboration. They include partnerships from pharmaceutical companies with government organizations, non-profit foundations and academic research centers.

Precompetitive research partnerships can be difficult to manage owing to the size and bureaucratic nature of large research partners. At times, there are legal challenges involving intellectual property rights that are often difficult to overcome. Umbrella initiatives provide the framework in which to negotiate specific networked projects under a defined theme.

There are several such truly public private initiatives. They focus on specific research processes such as biomarkers, adverse events and medicines. At this level of partnership not only are academic, CROs, biobanks, pharmaceutical and biotechnology efforts involved, regulatory bodies and other not-for-profit foundations and international research funders take part in the creation of the governance and financing infrastructure.

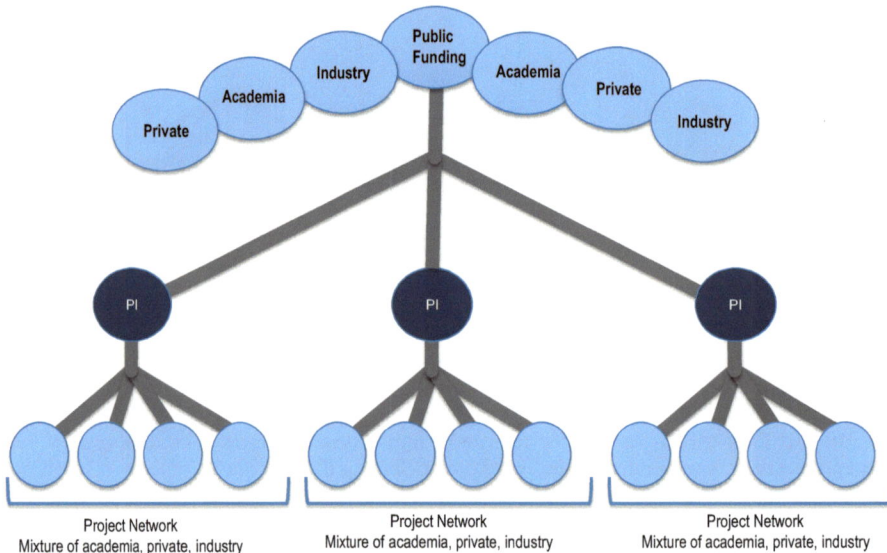

Fig (6). The umbrella initiative is a consortium of consortia that provides the governance and financial cover for the development of objective specific consortia in which the biobanks play a significant role.

The Innovative Medicines Initiative (IMI)

Perhaps one of the best examples of these umbrella initiatives for public private collaboration is the Innovative Medicines Initiative [62]. The IMI is Europe's largest public-private initiative, aiming to speed up the development of better, safer and more effective medicines for patients through a public-private partnership (PPP). IMI supports collaborative research projects and builds networks of industrial and academic experts to boost pharmaceutical innovation in Europe. It facilitates collaboration between the key players involved in healthcare research, including universities, the pharmaceutical and other industries, small and medium-sized enterprises (SMEs), patient organizations, and medicines regulators. IMI is a joint undertaking between the European Union and the European Federation of Pharmaceutical Industries and Associations (EFPIA) [63]. These have each contributed approximately 50% of budget for projects under this initiative. EFPIA companies and other Associated Partners do not receive EU funding, but contribute to the projects 'in kind', for example by donating their researchers' time or providing access to research facilities or resources [64]. IMI is a novel way of working that is radically changing the shape of the pharmaceutical research and development (R&D) landscape with more than 50 research projects funded, each with collaborations from academia, industry, SMEs and biobanks.

Ticking All The Boxes

Collaborations of this type remove the pain of finding the right form of collaboration in a specific research project. Having created the form and format, they provide the tools to help address the issues, such as IP, that continue to be stumbling blocks to successful collaborations. They also provide an arena for groups to find other partners to create projects for financing under the initiative. All potential players in research from patients to regulators are considered in microenvironment. Consideration is also given to SMEs to assist them to become part of the process.

These initiatives are different from framework programs in that they are more hands-on, compelling the partners, regardless of their culture, to adhere to a goal oriented project management. Partners must sit down together to plan and execute the research. While biobanks are specifically mentioned in these initiatives, these are not biobank specific PPPs. Biobanks cannot operate in an exclusive environment as they form part of the infrastructure on which research is constructed and are therefore an integral part of these initiatives. These initiatives serve biobanks well as they help put them in touch with a larger research and private industry community. While this is not a perfect world, it is certainly an attractive microenvironment for collaboration.

TURNING THE TABLES

More than perhaps anyone, pharmaceutical companies have had the opportunity to create biobanks of both biological materials and information collected through the recruitment of patients and collaboration with physicians during clinical trials. As such, they have the opportunity to make available their vast collections for academic research. Research departments within bio-industry companies believe that biobanks and the molecular information generated from them are outside the competitive realm and have the opportunity to demonstrate their willingness to share not only their incredible biobank resources but also their expertise. Some of these companies have begun finding ways to make these collections available to the entire research community - public and private alike.

Cancer Cell Line Encyclopedia (CCLE)

The Cancer Cell Line Encyclopedia (CCLE) project(8) is a collaboration between the Broad Institute, and the Novartis Institute for Biomedical Research and the Genomics Institute of the Novartis Research Foundation to conduct a detailed genetic and pharmacologic characterization of a large panel of human cancer models, to develop integrated computational analyses that link distinct pharmacologic vulnerabilities to genomic patterns and to translate cell line integrative genomics into cancer patient stratification. The CCLE provides public access to genomic data, analysis and visualization for about 1000 cell lines [66, 67].

This is an interesting turn about from the usual model of collaboration that sees the public partner as the one providing the biological materials and data. It is a model that fits into the model of expert centers but in an inverse mode where the private industrial partner is the one that is providing the data rather than in the classic model where a public entity provides the samples and associated data and the non-profit provides the expertise to provide the analytical data.

There are many such examples of industry sharing not only their research databases but also making their samples available to the general research community. This bodes well for new models of collaboration that go beyond focusing on samples and the data.

Academic Drug Discovery Centers

Academic drug Discovery Centers are, in a sense, spin-offs in reverse where industry forms an academic unit affiliated to a university [11, 68]. It is a model that approaches the best of both worlds, as it contains the organization of industry with the spirit and intellectual curiosity of academia [69]. This is the latest model of public private partnerships and an interesting area for biobank involvement. As they are a miniature of old pharmaceutical models with capability for molecular drug discovery they comprise all phases of the research path and as such need the biobank facility upon which to drive the research. As these academic drug discovery centers tend to be formed under a thematic scheme (cancer, infectious diseases, cardiovascular), for the integrated biobank they could be seen function as a mixture of the public-private model combined with the expert center. Merck and Pfizer are among the pharmaceutical companies that have set up academic drug discovery centers.

Academic Drug Discovery Consortium (ADDC)

A number of these centers have moved from a single structure to a networked or consortium structure and created the Academic Drug Discovery Consortium, whose goal is to build a collaborative network among the growing number of university-led drug discovery centers and programs. The consortium has nearly 1400 members and 130 drug discovery centers and its representational make-up is half academia and one quarter biotech/pharma and the rest comprised of government and philanthropic foundations (9).

THE WAY FORWARD

Biobanking is a relatively new multi-disciplinary activity much like the worlds from which it retrieves its samples. It functions on the border between diagnostics and patient care. Similarly, industry has been working in R&D for many years. Operating in a time sensitive commercial world, it has been working to strict time-lines and managing its investments and activities very well. Both academia and industry have a wealth of knowledge and experiences to share. This is a potential area of collaboration. To date, the only platforms for these experiences to be shared in an educational manner are through societies and associations [70]. However, some of the larger consortiums and networks indicated in this chapter have initiated Education and Training (E&T) programs [6]. One example is the ADDC presented previously that has provided access to training materials (presentations, videos, electronic books) in a modularized format. The IMI has gone one further and created an opportunity for financed collaborative PPP training programs. To date they focus on pharmaceutical training, safety sciences, and therapeutic innovation. However, as biobanks become more involved in these collaborative research projects and awareness of the importance of the biobank for reproducibility and pre-clinical validation increases, collaborative E&T programs on biobanking and the use of samples for molecular characterization can also be initiated.

CONCLUDING REMARKS

It is a somewhat predictable exercise to speak of biobanks in terms of samples and data and to speak of industry in terms of commerce and profit. Biobanks have been performing bio-specimen research and have invaluable information to inform correct bio-specimen characterization for biomarker evaluation. Academia has the mission of educating, providing tools for this education and integrating this with ground breaking research of the basic and translational variety. Industry has historically been more alert to changes in the healthcare system, as it must be to innovate, and therefore has the ability to inform research. Innovative technologies for molecular sequencing and metabolomics together with growing biospecimen resources have created the environment where biobanks, academia and industry can and must work together to develop the potential for discovery of new biomarkers and therapeutic targets this mass of information provides. This means that models for partnerships must continue to evolve to permit each collaborator to contribute and make good on the promise of truly personalized medicine.

CONFLICT OF INTEREST

The authors confirm that they have no conflict of interest to declare for this publication.

ACKNOWLEDGEMENT

ARC-Net Biobank has been partially funded by Italian Ministry of Health and Regione Veneto Public Funds.

REFERENCES

[1] Lengauer C, Diaz LA Jr, Saha S. Cancer drug discovery through collaboration. Nat Rev Drug Discov 2005; 4(5): 375-80.
[http://dx.doi.org/10.1038/nrd1722] [PMID: 15864266]

[2] Ledford H. Drug buddies. Nature 2011; 474(7352): 433-4.
[http://dx.doi.org/10.1038/474433a] [PMID: 21697923]

[3] Bravo E, Calzolari A, De Castro P, *et al.* Developing a guideline to standardize the citation of bioresources in journal articles (CoBRA). BMC Med 2015; 13: 33.
[http://dx.doi.org/10.1186/s12916-015-0266-y] [PMID: 25855867]

[4] Pronk JT, Lee SY, Lievense J, *et al.* How to set up collaborations between academia and industrial biotech companies. Nat Biotechnol 2015; 33(3): 237-40.
[http://dx.doi.org/10.1038/nbt.3171] [PMID: 25748909]

[5] Caulfield T, Burningham S, Joly Y, *et al.* A review of the key issues associated with the commercialization of biobanks. J Law Biosci 2014; 1(1): 94-110.
[http://dx.doi.org/10.1093/jlb/lst004] [PMID: 27774156]

[6] Rosenblatt M. How academia and the pharmaceutical industry can work together: the presidents lecture, annual meeting of the American Thoracic Society, San Francisco, California. Ann Am Thorac Soc 2013; 10(1): 31-8.
[http://dx.doi.org/10.1513/AnnalsATS.201209-075PS] [PMID: 23509330]

[7] Prinz F, Schlange T, Asadullah K. Believe it or not: how much can we rely on published data on potential drug targets? Nat Rev Drug Discov 2011; 10(9): 712.
[http://dx.doi.org/10.1038/nrd3439-c1] [PMID: 21892149]

[8] Jasny BR, Chin G, Chong L, Vignieri S. Data replication & reproducibility. Again, and again, and

again.... Introduction. Science 2011; 334(6060): 1225.
[http://dx.doi.org/10.1126/science.334.6060.1225] [PMID: 22144612]

[9] Caulfield T, Harmon SH, Joly Y. Open science *versus* commercialization: a modern research conflict? Genome Med 2012; 4(2): 17.
[http://dx.doi.org/10.1186/gm316] [PMID: 22369790]

[10] Lei Z, Juneja R, Wright BD. Patents *versus* patenting: implications of intellectual property protection for biological research. Nat Biotechnol 2009; 27(1): 36-40.
[http://dx.doi.org/10.1038/nbt0109-36] [PMID: 19131994]

[11] Tralau-Stewart CJ, Wyatt CA, Kleyn DE, Ayad A. Drug discovery: new models for industry-academic partnerships. Drug Discov Today 2009; 14(1-2): 95-101.
[http://dx.doi.org/10.1016/j.drudis.2008.10.003] [PMID: 18992364]

[12] Yuille M, Dixon K, Platt A, *et al.* The UK DNA banking network: a fair access biobank. Cell Tissue Bank 2010; 11(3): 241-51.
[http://dx.doi.org/10.1007/s10561-009-9150-3] [PMID: 19672698]

[13] Heinemann JA. Funding for knowledge-sake - Letter. Drug Discov Today 2000; 5(6): 222-3.
[http://dx.doi.org/10.1016/S1359-6446(00)01510-5] [PMID: 10825725]

[14] Kozlowski RZ. Industrial-academic collaboration: a bridge too far? Drug Discov Today 1999; 4(11): 487-9.
[http://dx.doi.org/10.1016/S1359-6446(99)01416-6] [PMID: 10529764]

[15] Schachter B. Partnering with the professor. Nat Biotechnol 2012; 30(10): 944-52.
[http://dx.doi.org/10.1038/nbt.2385] [PMID: 23051810]

[16] Geary J, Jardine CG, Guebert J, Bubela T. Access and benefits sharing of genetic resources and associated traditional knowledge in northern Canada: understanding the legal environment and creating effective research agreements. Int J Circumpolar Health 2013; 72: 72.
[http://dx.doi.org/10.3402/ijch.v72i0.21351] [PMID: 23986896]

[17] Evers K, Forsberg JS, Eliason JF. What are your views on commercialization of tissues for research? Biopreserv Biobank 2012; 10(6): 476-8.
[http://dx.doi.org/10.1089/bio.2012.1062] [PMID: 24845132]

[18] Lemke AA, Wolf WA, Hebert-Beirne J, Smith ME. Public and biobank participant attitudes toward genetic research participation and data sharing. Public Health Genomics 2010; 13(6): 368-77.
[http://dx.doi.org/10.1159/000276767] [PMID: 20805700]

[19] Haddow G, Laurie G, Cunningham-Burley S, Hunter KG. Tackling community concerns about commercialisation and genetic research: a modest interdisciplinary proposal. Soc Sci Med 2007; 64(2): 272-82.
[http://dx.doi.org/10.1016/j.socscimed.2006.08.028] [PMID: 17050056]

[20] Hansson MG. Building on relationships of trust in biobank research. J Med Ethics 2005; 31(7): 415-8.
[http://dx.doi.org/10.1136/jme.2004.009456] [PMID: 15994363]

[21] Hoeyer K. Trust in Biobanking. springer 2012.

[22] Critchley C, Nicol D, Otlowski M. The impact of commercialisation and genetic data sharing arrangements on public trust and the intention to participate in biobank research. Public Health Genomics 2015; 18(3): 160-72.
[http://dx.doi.org/10.1159/000375441] [PMID: 25790760]

[23] Clemence MG N, Shah J, Swiecicka J, *et al.* Wellcome Trust Monitor Wave 2. Wellcome Trust. Ipsos MORI 2013.

[24] Critchley CRaN D. D. Understanding the Impact of Commercialization on Public Support for Scientific Research: is It about the Funding Source or the Organization Conducting the Research. Science 2004.

[25] Pullman D, Etchegary H, Gallagher K, *et al.* Personal privacy, public benefits, and biobanks: a conjoint analysis of policy priorities and public perceptions. Genetics in medicine : official journal of the American College of Medical Genetics 2012; 14(2): 229-35.
[http://dx.doi.org/10.1038/gim.0b013e31822e578f]

[26] Ursin LO. Privacy and property in the biobank context. HEC forum : an interdisciplinary journal on hospitals' ethical and legal issues 2010; 22(3): 211-4.
[http://dx.doi.org/10.1007/s10730-010-9138-1]

[27] Wolf SM, Crock BN, Van Ness B, *et al.* Managing incidental findings and research results in genomic research involving biobanks and archived data sets. Genetics in medicine : official journal of the American College of Medical Genetics 2012; 14(4): 361-84.
[http://dx.doi.org/10.1038/gim.2012.23]

[28] Yüzbaşıoğlu A, Özgüç M. Biobanking: sample acquisition and quality assurance for omics research. N Biotechnol 2013; 30(3): 339-42.
[http://dx.doi.org/10.1016/j.nbt.2012.11.016] [PMID: 23183539]

[29] http://www.icgc.org.

[30] Hudson TJ, Anderson W, Artez A, *et al.* International network of cancer genome projects. Nature 2010; 464(7291): 993-8.
[http://dx.doi.org/10.1038/nature08987] [PMID: 20393554]

[31] Hughes SE, Barnes RO, Watson PH. Biospecimen use in cancer research over two decades. Biopreserv Biobank 2010; 8(2): 89-97.
[http://dx.doi.org/10.1089/bio.2010.0005] [PMID: 24845937]

[32] Heeney C, Hawkins N, de Vries J, Boddington P, Kaye J. Assessing the privacy risks of data sharing in genomics. Public Health Genomics 2011; 14(1): 17-25.
[http://dx.doi.org/10.1159/000294150] [PMID: 20339285]

[33] Ragin C, Park JY. Biospecimens, biobanking and global cancer research collaborations. Ecancermedicalscience 2014; 8: 454.
[PMID: 25228910]

[34] Kling J. Biotechs follow big pharma lead back into academia. Nat Biotechnol 2011; 29(7): 555-6.
[http://dx.doi.org/10.1038/nbt0711-555] [PMID: 21747364]

[35] Lench N. A meeting of the minds: working with academia, http://www.pharmafile.com/news/meeting-minds-working-academia. Pharmafocus 2007.

[36] MEIJER IM-G J, Mattsson P. Networked Research Infrastructures and their governance: The case of Biobanking. Sci Public Policy 2012; 39.

[37] (Standardisaton and improvement of genetic Pre-nalytical tools and procedures for *In-vitro* DIAgnostics, http://www.spidia.eu/.

[38] Tops BB, Normanno N, Kurth H, *et al.* Development of a semi-conductor sequencing-based panel for genotyping of colon and lung cancer by the Onconetwork consortium. BMC Cancer 2015; 15: 26.
[http://dx.doi.org/10.1186/s12885-015-1015-5] [PMID: 25637035]

[39] MAGDALENO SM. The OncoNetwork Consortium: a global collaborative research study on the development and verification of an Ion AmpliSeq™ RNA Lung Fusion Panel. Cancer Research 2014; 74(19 Supplement): 3573-4.
[http://dx.doi.org/10.1186/s12885-015-1015-5] [PMID: 25637035]

[40] Tactacan CM, Chang DK, Cowley MJ, *et al.* RON is not a prognostic marker for resectable pancreatic cancer. BMC Cancer 2012; 12: 395.
[http://dx.doi.org/10.1186/1471-2407-12-395] [PMID: 22958871]

[41] Turner AD-F C, Murtagh MJ. Biobank Economics and the "Commercialization Problem". Spontaneous Generations 2013; 7(1).

[42]   Nussbeck SY, Rabone M, Benson EE, Droege G, Mackenzie-Dodds J, Lawlor RT. Life in dataoutcome of a multi-disciplinary, interactive biobanking conference session on sample data. Biopreserv Biobank 2016; 14(1): 56-64.
[http://dx.doi.org/10.1089/bio.2015.0061] [PMID: 26808538]

[43]   http://www.lifandis.com/.

[44]   http://www.biobankdenmark.dk/About the Biobank/The Biobank Organization.aspx.

[45]   http://www.nordforsk.org/en.

[46]   http://www.ntnu.no/biobanknorge/nordic-biobank-network.

[47]   Baker M. Big biotech buys iconic genetics firm. Nature 2012; 492(7429): 321.
[http://dx.doi.org/10.1038/492321a]

[48]   Kaiser J. Big biotech buys iconic genetics firm, http://www.technologyreview.com/news/536096/genome-study-predicts-dna-of-the-whole-of-iceland/.492(7429). 2002.

[49]   Winickoff DE, Winickoff RN. The charitable trust as a model for genomic biobanks. N Engl J Med 2003; 349(12): 1180-4.
[http://dx.doi.org/10.1056/NEJMsb030036] [PMID: 13679534]

[50]   Ruzzenente A, Fassan M, Conci S, *et al.* Cholangiocarcinoma heterogeneity revealed by multigene mutational profiling: clinical and prognostic relevance in surgically resected patients. Ann Surg Oncol 2015; 23(5): 1699-707.
[PMID: 26717940]

[51]   http://www.wellcome.ac.uk/.

[52]   http://www.mrc.ac.uk/index.htm.

[53]   http://www.dh.gov.uk/en/index.htm.

[54]   http://home.scotland.gov.uk/home.

[55]   Huzair FP, Biobank TU. Consequences for commons and innovation. Sci Public Policy 2012; 39.

[56]   Gomez-Rubio P, Zock JP, Rava M, *et al.* Reduced risk of pancreatic cancer associated with asthma and nasal allergies. Gut 2015; 66(2): 314-22.
[PMID: 26628509]

[57]   Winickoff DE. Partnership in U.K. Biobank: a third way for genomic property? The Journal of law, medicine & ethics: a journal of the American Society of Law. Med Ethics (Burlingt, Mass) 2007; 35(3): 440-56.

[58]   Hofman P, Bréchot C, Zatloukal K, Dagher G, Clément B. Public-private relationships in biobanking: a still underestimated key component of open innovation. Virchows Arch 2014; 464(1): 3-9.
[http://dx.doi.org/10.1007/s00428-013-1524-z] [PMID: 24337181]

[59]   van Ommen GJ, Törnwall O, Bréchot C, *et al.* BBMRI-ERIC as a resource for pharmaceutical and life science industries: the development of biobank-based Expert Centres. Eur J Hum Genet 2015; 23(7): 893-900.
[http://dx.doi.org/10.1038/ejhg.2014.235] [PMID: 25407005]

[60]   http://www.excemet.org/.

[61]   Carotenuto D, Luchinat C, Marcon G, Rosato A, Turano P. The da vinci european bioBank: a metabolomics-driven infrastructure. J Pers Med 2015; 5(2): 107-19.
[http://dx.doi.org/10.3390/jpm5020107] [PMID: 25913579]

[62]   https://www.imi.europa.eu/.

[63]   http://imi.efpia.eu/.

[64]   Funding Model IM. https://www.imi.europa.eu/content/imi-funding-model.

[65]   http://www.csrwire.com/press_releases/33936-Novartis-Launches-the-Cancer-Cell-Line-Encyclopedia
        -CCLE-to-Catalogue-World-s-Cancer-Cell-Lines.

[66]   http://www.cbioportal.org/study?id=cellline_ccle_broad - summary.

[67]   http://portals.broadinstitute.org/ccle/home.

[68]   Frye S, Crosby M, Edwards T, Juliano R. US academic drug discovery. Nat Rev Drug Discov 2011;
        10(6): 409-10.
        [http://dx.doi.org/10.1038/nrd3462] [PMID: 21629285]

[69]   Slusher BS, Conn PJ, Frye S, Glicksman M, Arkin M. Bringing together the academic drug discovery
        community. Nat Rev Drug Discov 2013; 12(11): 811-2.
        [http://dx.doi.org/10.1038/nrd4155] [PMID: 24172316]

[70]   http://www.addconsortium.org/about-landing.php.

CHAPTER 3

Quality Management System for Research Biobanks: a Tool to Incentivize Public-Private Partnerships

Elena Bravo* and Mariarosaria Napolitano

Research Coordination and Support Service, Istituto Superiore di Sanità (National Institute of Health), Rome, Italy

Abstract: Biospecimens are essential raw materials for the advancement of applied biotechnology. Awareness of the importance of sharing biospecimens has increased in recent years and biobanking activities have facilitated access to them. However, the sharing of such samples for Research & Development could be considerably improved if there were a recognised global agreement about the standard by which to compare their quality.

The Organization for Standardization (ISO) is the internationally recognised body that provides guidelines and defines specifications to ensure standardisation of materials, processes and products. The working group two (WG2) of the ISO Technical Committee (TC) 276 established by the ISO on Biotechnology is dedicated to Biobanking. The aim of this working group is to establish sets of standards that apply to the biobanking field, to include human, animal, plant and microorganism samples, thus ensuring that they are of appropriate quality. The availability of worldwide recognized policies and procedures will support access and exchange of samples and related data, giving a major impetus to global use of bioresources for market application.

The standard set, which will be based on existing documents and guidelines, will be the foundation of a quality management system (QMS) specifically for biobanking. ISO QMS would enable the establishment of ad hoc global certification that products, processes and/or services conform to relevant standards, technical specifications and guidelines.

Keywords: Accreditation, Biobanking, Bioeconomy, Biological resources centres (brc), Bioresource, Biospecimen, Biotechnology, Certification, Guidelines, Harmonization, International Standard (is), International standard organization (iso), Market, Personalized medicine, Quality Control (qc), Quality Management

---

* **Corresponding author Elena Bravo:** Research Coordination and Support Service, Istituto Superioredi Sanità (National Institute of Health), Rome, Italy; Tel: +39 06 4990 3061; Email: elena.bravo@iss.it

Elena Salvaterra and Julie Corfield (Eds.)
All rights reserved-© 2017 Bentham Science Publishers

System (QMS), Repository, Standardization, Technical committee 2761.

1. QUALITY REQUIREMENTS: A BRIDGE BETWEEN PUBLIC AND PRIVATE SECTORS

Public and private sectors are often based on different principles and language. Two of the critical issues in the establishment of Public Private partnership (PPP) in biobanking are represented by a common ground for defining biospecimens and for comparison of available biological resources. Standardization of requirements for the quality of biospecimens would provide a useful tools to overcome some of the major difficulties in facilitating fruitful exchange of samples and data for the development of both research and market applications.

1.1. From the Roots of Quality to Management System Standard(s) [MSS]

Quality is an historic concept which has its roots in the late 13th century, when craftsmen began organizing into guilds responsible with strict rules regulating the quality of products and services This approach was followed until the early 19th century. During the 20th century, the idea of Total Quality Management began to emerge as we know today, and for the first time statistical theory was applied to product quality control (QC). The early work of Shewhart in drafting statistical methods for process control was later developed by Deming in the Plan-Do-Check-Act (PDCA) theory [1]. The four phases in the PDCA Cycle involve:

- Identifying and analyzing the problem (Plan)
- Developing and testing a potential solution (Do)
- Measuring how effective the test solution was, and analyzing whether it could be improved in any way (Check)
- Implementing the improved solution fully (Act)

Plan–do–check–act is an iterative four-step management method used in business for the control and continuous improvement of processes and products. The early work of Shewhart and Deming [2] constitutes much of what today comprises the theory of statistical process control. However, there was little use of these techniques in manufacturing companies until the late 1940's.

During its history, quality management (QM) has gone through numerous changes, but the aim remains the same: to improve customer satisfaction. Therefore, the quality of a product may be defined as "its ability to fulfil the customer's needs and expectations". However, quality needs to be defined by criteria which vary from product to product. For "concrete items", the term quality applies and refers to the degree to which a set of inherent characteristics fulfil a set of requirements. For mechanical or electronic products, quality requirements include performance, reliability, safety and appearance, while quality standards for pharmaceutical products need to involve physical and chemical characteristics, medicinal effect, toxicity, taste and shelf life [3]. Often it is a chain of processes (procedures to transform inputs into outputs) that deliver a product or the final object. Thus, a "process approach" is a management strategy that allows the management and control of the processes that make up the organization. A management system may be restricted to a specific function or section of an organization, it may include the entire organization or it may even cut across several organizations. There are many types of management system including, for example, environmental management systems, disaster mana-gement systems, risk management systems *etc*. Many of these include a quality management system (QMS).

Thus, a QMS is a set of interrelated or interacting components that organizations/ industries/bodies use to formulate quality policies and quality objectives and to establish the processes that are needed to ensure that policies are followed and objectives are achieved. The QMS involve human and material resources, structures, organization, plans, processes and tracking. In other words, a QMS is nothing more than good business sense and is the establishment of policies, processes and controls that can impact on the organization's ability to meet customer requirements and there is a big effort to apply it also in biobanking [4].

The quality policy and objectives of QMS are achieved through quality assurance (QA) and QC, which, respectively, focus on the processes through which the product is produced and on the product itself.

A QMS is linked to the important concept of the external recognition of quality, which relates to requirements specified in Licenses to Trade, guidelines, specified customer requirements, and the chosen management system standard(s) [MSS].

1.2. Biobanking Worldwide: State of Art

Biological materials, including samples from humans, animals, plants and microorganisms and/or their derivatives are a major resource for the advancement of food industries, human and animal health and Research & Development (R&D) in life sciences. Activities related to sampling, cataloguing, studying, storing and distributing biospecimens are known as biobanking. In the last decade biobanking has spread widely in terms of both of new sites and developing solutions for the exploitation of sector potentialities. This increased global interest has produced many studies concerning biobanking activities, management and networking, and also related issues including legal, ethical, quantity *vs* quality aspects of biological resources and their sustainability [5].

Until the turn of the millennium, most biobanks were located in North America and Europe, but the biobank landscape is changing rapidly worldwide. There are now several biospecimens networks operative in Australia, mostly set up in the last decade as non profit organization funded through Australian governmental and public/advocacy organizations [6].

The Asian Consortium for the Conservation and Sustainable Use of Microbial Resources [7] established in 2004, aims to promote collaboration among government or public organizations in Asian countries for the purposes of enhancing conservation and sustainable use of microbial resources. The 13 members (Cambodia, China, India, Indonesia, Japan, Korea, Laos, Malaysia, Mongolia, Myanmar, Philippines, Thailand and Vietnam) of the ACM Consortium are government or public institutes, or universities actively engaged in developing microbial resources characteristic for each country and in establishing international standards for biological material transfer and benefit-sharing.

In recent years, in China several initiatives have aimed to set up a biobanking national network. To support both scientific research and commercial applications, the China National Genebank (CNGB) [8] based in Shenzhen has provided a platform for information sharing and exchange of materials and "omics" data since 2008. Several developing countries such as Gambia, Jordan, Mexico and South Africa have also established their own biobanks and biobanking networks [9].

1.3. Quality and Biobanking

The growing awareness and understanding of the importance of biobanking have made it increasingly clear that there are major obstacles to the use of samples in partnership. These relate to the availability of good samples which can be used to achieve solid results and to obtaining the appropriate permissions for their use in collaborative studies. Thus, much biobanking constructive work has focused on developing appropriate policies, initiatives and guidelines to improve sample quality and quantity. Concepts related to the potential economic impact of producing high quality tools and providing access to quality resources (like samples, healthcare databases, genetic databases, *etc.*) have been defined elsewhere [10, 11].

In parallel, much effort in Western countries has been dedicated to the analysis of ethical and legal issues, such as informed consent, material transfer agreements, transboundary use,data protection, ownership, commercialization and public participation [12]. Indeed, Citizens, as donors or patients [13], are increasingly aware that they are actively participating in the development of biobanking.

Furthermore, disease-focused foundations, advocacy organizations and commercial entities which want to develop new therapies and diagnostic tools for diseases are becoming an important source of capital to generate new biobanking initiatives [14].

Social attention and media interest has grown and given rise to optimism, but also for our health and aging but also concerns for safety issues. Although public knowledge has increased to a different extent in different countries, the discussion about ethical, regulatory and legal issues has moved from a local to a global level. Due to local culture, religious beliefs and different perception of behavioural fairness and ethics, the proliferation of biobanks in low- and middle- income countries [15] new ethical, cross-border and benefit-sharing issues have arisen which are not found in other areas of human research [16, 17]. These concerns have a negative impact on international research collaborations, thus there is need to develop a global governance framework to guarantee equity, fairness and justice in biobank collaboration between developing and developed countries [18].

To implement shared applicable solutions to maximize the utilization of biobanking resources, regional and transnational networking initiatives and valuable worldwide grids are continuing to develop.

In Europe, biobanking has been identified as an area of strategic interest by the European Strategy Forum on Research Infrastructures (ESFRI), and the legal consortium named "Biobanking and Biomolecular Resources Research Infrastructure" (BBMRI-ERIC) has been established [19]. BBMRI-ERIC is a bio-medical and life science infrastructure for the sustainable storage and dissemination of banked human samples and associated data. Driven by the opportunity to participate in BBMRI, the European countries set up national infrastructures (national nodes) and made considerable efforts to establish national, regional as well as population *vs* disease oriented networks [20].

International initiatives, such as the Public Population Project in Genomics and Society [21], the International Society for Biological and Environmental Repositories (ISBER) [22] and the International Agency for Research on Cancer (IARC) [23], have offered governance structures models, best practices and guidelines to promote the internationalization and standardization of biobanks.

All these documents have given an impetus to efforts to harmonize and to find a common consensus about biobanking activities. The global interest resulted in a number of successes which can be summarized in a huge change in the cultural approach to biobanking activities and increased capability (technical, ethical-legal, social and economic) to face biobanking challenges.

Large numbers of valuable materials were collected, and at least 80 different guidelines, best practice and harmonisation studies results have been produced. A list of the most used guideline implemented both at national and international level is available from P3G website [24].

The analysis of these guidelines shows certain degree of heterogeneity in term of principles and activities addressed. Furthermore, some area of biobanking remain outside any of these guidelines. Thus, in spite of the rapidly growing interest and attention [25, 26], there is still a lack of clear definition of the quality requirements for biospecimens, Benefit-sharing issues in cross-border flows of samples remains additional obstacles to international research and applicative collaboration. In this scenario it is not surprising that access to the samples is still a major area which needs to be improved, and that public biobanks still remain an underused source of biospecimens for public research and, even more, for the development of processes and products by private companies [27].

In other worlds, at all levels there is growing evidence of the necessity of recognised standards to make the exchange of quality assured bioresources easier, safer, and faster. Thanks to available and reliable biological resources the markets and the research became flourishing.

A legal tool by which information is validated and transmitted today is the certification. In many sectors certification schemes are used in place of public control systems. Certification requires a valid and recognized set of reference norms.

To respond to the lack of global recognized standards for biological specimens, a working group (WG) of the Technical Committee (TC) 276 on Biotechnology, set up by the International Organization for Standardization (ISO) [28], has been dedicated to the Biobanking.

2. STANDARD, CERTIFICATION AND ACCREDITATION

2.1. Formal Standard

The term "formal standard" is adopted only for specifications or requirements that have been approved by the national standard setting organization. Nowadays, there are a number of organizations devoted primarily to work to develop, promulgate and update standards that aim to meet the need of a large swath of potential adopters/users. These include governmental or treaty organizations, nongovernmental organizations, and organizations that are either specialized in standardization or involved also in other activities. The largest and most consolidated organizations are the International Organization for Standardization

(ISO), the International Electrotechnical Commission (IEC), and the International Telecommunication Union (ITU). These bodies that develop standards used globally and have established standards covering almost every possible topic. ISO and IEC are both private, voluntary organizations whose members are National Standards Bodies (NSBs), one per member economy. The International Standard (IS) delivered by the ISO Technical Committee (TC) express the consensus reached among the NSBs, which represent social and economic interests at the international level. IS can take many forms comprising standards, norms, technical reports, guidelines, test methods, codes of practice, guideline standards and MSS. Thus, ISO MSSs provide a model to follow when setting up and operating a management system with a definition of QMS required for planning, developing and executing activities/service in a core business area.

With regard to their application, these standards are voluntary recognized by most of the world's countries and most of the global standard certifications are based on the ISO rules. However, the ISO norms do not supersede or substitute any applicable legal requirements. Through the application of national and international standards, government, procurers and consumers can have confidence in the calibration and test results, inspection reports and certifications provided. In response to the application of an ISO norms a firm can be certified according to a defined IS.

2.2. Certification and Accreditation

Certification and accreditation are two terms, sometimes, (incorrectly) used interchangeably, but they are dissimilar concepts, although their exact definition depend on the geographic location, language and thematic environment in which they are used.

In general, accreditation (called in some case licencing) is the procedure by which an authoritative body/organization gives formal recognition that a body or person is competent to carry out specific tasks. These tasks include testing, calibration, certification, and inspection. Certification, on the other hand, is a procedure which certifies that a product, process, service or person conforms to specified requirements in specific areas. Certification may be mandatory, in which case it is carried out according to local/ international law, or voluntary where a third party provides the written assurance and is adopted by companies to demonstrate the performance of their organizations or products.

Government/institutional accreditation for a biobank is, for instance, the recognition of compliance with requirements established from either regional (regional accreditation) or national bodies (national accreditation). These requirements may include parameters relating to the structure, the type of personnel and the quality system. Thus, the accreditation is the authorization of the activity provided by the super-ordinated Authority or a local institutional recognition of the excellence of scientific work.

Several other accreditation processes may coexist. For instance, accreditation promoted by professional associations/organizations/societies and academies. These are generally for professionals/Institutions in their performance of specific activities. It is noteworthy that both institutional and professional accreditation is awarded by institutions or bodies that retain functional relationship with the accredited facilities (*i.e.* independence is not guaranteed).

To ensure the independence of standard setting and evaluation, the ISO's norms certification schemes appoint a third-party accreditation body to assess the suitability and qualification of certification bodies for their system. In order to guarantee users of the competence and impartiality of the body accredited, a unique and independent National Accreditation Body (NAB) have been established in each country with the primary purpose of ensuring that conformity assessment bodies are subject to oversight by an authoritative body. The accreditation hierarchy is overseen by the International Accreditation Forum (IAF) [29] and the European co-operation for Accreditation (EA) [30]. The NABs that are member of IAF [29] signed a mutual recognition agreement (Multilateral Recognition Arrangements) which recognize the equivalence of other members' accreditations to their own because they have undergone equivalent stringent peer evaluations.

In Europe, in full compliance with the regulation of the European Parliament and Commission n° 765 of July 9, 2008 every European country established a unique NAB, officially recognized by their national Governments, to assess and verify organizations that carry out evaluation services such as certification, verification, inspection, testing and calibration. NABs are non-profit-distributing organizations that provide these conformity assessment services in compliance with the international standards such as the series ISO 17000 and of the guides and the harmonized series of European norms EN 45000. Accreditation by the NAB and/or certification body accredited by the NAB is able to thoroughly assess clients against these requirements and issue certificates in an impartial manner. Thus, in certification clients should always ensure their selected Certification Body has been accredited by the NAB.

Certification process according to ISO's norms is used for verifying that personnel, objects, or organizations have adequate credentials to practice certain disciplines, as well as for verifying that products meet certain requirements, and is the confirmation that the certified client/product is in line with a set of requirements, provided by the ISO. However, certification makes no judgment about how similar products compare and certification does not aim to indicate which product is best.

The certification procedure by the accredited body is followed by the quality audit which is the process of systematic examination of a quality system carried out by an internal or external quality auditor or an audit team. Audits are an essential part of the management system approach as they enable the client to check how far their achievements meet their objectives and show conformity to the standard. The quality audit is an integral part of organization's QMS and is a key element in the certification ISO. Audits must be independent and evidence must be evaluated objectively to determine how well audit criteria are being met ISO 19011:2011 provides specific guidance on internal and external management system audits.

3. ISO/TC276 BIOTECHNOLOGY

In the early 1970s, with the development of innovative biotechnology, it became necessary to address the issue of quality in that field. According to the Organisation for Economic Co-operation and Development (OECD), Biotechnology is defined as "The application of science and technology to living organisms, as well as parts, products and models thereof, to alter living or non-living materials for the production of knowledge, goods and services [31]". In other words, biotechnology builds on disciplines such as biology and biochemistry, but it requires specific knowledge derived from others, including physics, chemistry, engineering, materials science and computer science. New bioprocesses, which are additional to traditional biotechnology processes such as fermentation, mutation, and plant and animal hybridization, are more and more offering technical solutions, performance and capabilities to many different sectors, such as healthcare and medicine, agricultural and industrial production. Biotechnology terms defined according to OECD are reported in Table 1 [31].

The emerging "bioeconomy" promotes eco-sustainable production of renewable resources and their conversion into food, bio-based products, biofuels and bioenergy and contributes to a significant share of economic output. Biotechnology as a cross-sectional technology, has an important role in the bioeconomy playing a key part in the production of pharmaceuticals, agricultural chemicals,the value of which is estimated to grow to be 2.7% of global Gross Domestic Product by 2030 [32]. The applications of Biotechnology offer new opportunities to address many needs, and it is thus regarded as a major contributor to economic growth and job creation, public health, environmental protection and sustainable development [33]. This market for biotechnology is global and is continually evolving due to the vast number of new technologies being developed.

Table 1. Biotechnology terms defined according to OECD [31] definition according to OECD of common Biotechnology terms.

Category	
DNA / RNA	Genomics, pharmacogenomics, gene probes, genetic engineering, DNA/RNA sequencing/synthesis/amplification, gene expression profiling, and use of antisense technology.
Proteins and molecules	Sequencing/synthesis/engineering of proteins and peptides (including large molecule hormones); improved delivery methods for large molecule drugs; proteomics, protein isolation and purification, signaling, identification of cell receptors.
Cell and tissue culture and engineering	Cell and tissue culture, tissue engineering (including tissue scaffolds and biomedical engineering), cellular fusion, vaccine/immune stimulants, embryo manipulation.
Process biotechnology's	Fermentation using bioreactors, bioprocessing, bioleaching, biopulping, biobleaching, biodesulphurisation, bioremediation, biofiltration and phytoremediation.
Gene and RNA vectors	Gene therapy, viral vectors.
Bioinformatics	Construction of databases on genomes, protein sequences; modelling complex biological processes, including systems biology.
Nanobiotechnology	Applies the tools and processes of nano/micro fabrication to build devices for studying biosystems and applications in drug delivery, diagnostics *etc*.

The first aim of ISO standards is to responds to the need for companies to access new markets, facilitate free and fair global trade and to ensure that products and services are safe, reliable and of good quality. Biotechnology development is an engine and catalyst for investments and benefits. Furthermore, the Technical Management Board (TMB), the body responsible for the general management of the ISO technical committee structure and of their implementation, has recognized the existence of suitable commercial, regulatory and social environment conditions that would be supportive of further Biotechnology growth. This recognition has brought to the establishment of the TC276 Biotechnology.

There is, in fact, a great global interest in biotechnology and, so far, 25 countries are participating member of the committee and 14 countries take part as observer members. The secretariat is located in Germany (DIN, the German Institute for Standardization). The TC 276 Biotechnology is a horizontal committee cross cutting technology within many sectors and plays a key role in a multitude of processes and applications with the main objective of facilitating the exchange of goods and services through the elimination of technical barriers to trade [34]. The leading concept is that biotechnology standardization will aid growth in productivity by supporting innovation, value generation, compliance and regulation.

TC276 is organized in Working Groups (WGs) and each WG operates with a similar general methodological approach:

 i. A preliminary process of evaluation and comparison of existing standards to draw a picture of what is currently available, or already achieved
 ii. Identification of gaps and needs, considered to be a further early step
iii. Decision on work items to be addressed by the committee that primarily take into account the needs of businesses and the market
iv. Development of standards that do not conflict with any relevant existing national or regional statutory or regulatory requirements or guidelines
 v. Each phase of the work will take account of related committees and will collaborate with other organizations to avoid duplication and overlapping standardization activities

The TC276 recognizes that some biotech sectors are from the most highly regulated industries in the world, (*i.e:* processes in food, agriculture or medicinal products) and it will not address regulation in these fields unless specific gaps are identified.

The scope of the established ISO/TC276 [28] is standardization in the field of biotechnology processes and, so far, the following WGs have been activated:

• WG1: terms and definitions;
• WG2: biobanking;
• WG3: analytical methods;
• WG4:bioprocessing;
• WG5: data processing and integration.

WG1: Terms and definitions. The use of a harmonized vocabulary, which overcomes regional differences and translational difficulties, and different uses of scientific terms is essential to deliver set of norm which will be globally applied. WG1 is devoted to develop a compendium of biotechnology-related terms. The scope imposes a methodology of work closely collaborative with the other WGs and requires intensive cross- coordination activity. WG1 will work on identification of currently used national and international standards, guidelines and other relevant documents, as well as biotechnology-related terms and definitions. The expected outcome is a Technical Report which contains the foundation for the identification of gaps and needs in biotechnological terminology, and the definition of related terms. Initially, the work of WG1, where possible, will focus on harmonization rather than on standardization.

WG2: A package of IS in the Biobanking field including human, animal, plant and microorganism resources for R&D, but excluding therapeutic products, will be established. The activities of WG2 address the full series of regulatory and ethical requirements that biosample-based applications must fulfil to ensure environmental and human safety and the protection of rights during their development and before they are released into the market. WG2 is discussed in detail below.

WG3: Analytical methods. The scope of this WG is to develop standards for accurate, reproducible and robust measurement and analysis in support of biotechnologies. Development of analytical methods-related standards integrate the activities of WG2 and WG4. Deliverables will be a package of IS norms for biologically relevant molecules and entities, including nucleic acids, proteins, and cells. The standards developed will be mostly horizontal, as they are addressed to very specific issues. For particular applications in some industrial sectors standards will be vertical. So far some work items have been defined and specific norms on cell enumeration, nucleic acid quantification, nucleic acid sequencing, protein identification and quantification and cell characterization are expected to be the first deliverables of the WG3.

WG4: Bioprocessing. This WG will focus on processes and not on end uses. Fermentation, biocatalysis and, generally, the use of bacteria and/or enzymes to obtain different products or to control/maintain/optimize the rate of a machine or process, commonly referred as traditional biotechnology. Bioprocessing is a growth family of procedures (*i.e.* hybridization, cell/tissue culture, genetic and molecular engineering) at the base of expanding sectors such as, for instance, cell therapy bioprocessing, biopharmaceutical manufacturing. The aim of WG4 is to develop IS, technical reports and guidelines to give confidence to suppliers when developing or operating bioprocesses, and to users when products are put on the market or into a supply chain. WG4 has identified the primary 4 phases of bioprocessing that are in need of standardization:

1. Component materials control. WG4 will ensure criteria for the use of components and/or materials that ensure consistent and reproducible quality and the appropriate level of safety, including requirements in the choice of service providers and definition of contract manufacturers.
2. Bioreactor processes. Biotechnology processes need to operate under a specified degree of control. Control, maintenance and custody throughout the bioreactor processes lifecycle is another area that has been identified as in need of standardization. As a starting point, TG4 is considering how to develop standards or guidelines for bioprocessing of cells.
3. Product processing. A set of procedure will be dedicated to the procedures for collection, separation, purification and formulation/assembly of delivered products.

4. Handling, transportation and storage. Rules will be made available to ensure an appropriate distribution for the delivery of products.

WG5: Data processing and integration. The excellence of delivered biotech applications and of related research is strongly dependent on data quality. For instance, annotation linked to the samples and health file information are an integral part of the biobank patrimony. The standards expected to be delivered by WG5 will define/set norms for annotation, analysis, validation, comparability, exchange and integration of data. Some of the major objectives of this WG, have been already identified. Commonly recognized models which provide suitable formats for data is highly desirable. Building on the most common standards already in use, recommendations will be delivered for a structured and coherent formatting of life science data.

Data integration is also related to meta-data and how these data should be described, defining, in addition, their components and relationships. To produce guidelines on data integration, WG5 will produce standard workflows of data which will aid, for instance, in generating, formatting, defining, simulating and envisaging life computer models.

A WG6 Metrology, has been planned, but activities have not yet been started.

4. WG2 "BIOBANKING"

The establishment of a TC committee by ISO is strongly connected to the mission of ISO' norms which aims to facilitate trading and exchange of goods and services, supporting sustainable economic growth as well as to promote innovation and protect health, safety and the environment. Other criteria that should are used to define a targeted topic for the agenda of an ISO TC are: i. Global relevance; ii. Clear and understandable reasons for the necessity of such a standard; iii. Convincing reasoning also for people not involved in the sector; iv. A solid basis of knowledge in the target area.

The strategic plan [28] of the ISO TC276 provides an overview of the reasons for establishment of the TC on Biotechnology as well as the aim and methodology, which are summarized below.

4.1. Aim of WG2

The WG2 of TC276 will elaborate several sets of IS that apply to the biobanking field, including human, animal, plant and microorganism samples, to ensure appropriate quality of samples for R&D, but excluding therapeutic both application and products. The expected documents that take into account existing documents and guidelines, will state the requirements needed to ensure appropriate quality of the collections by implementing QM and QC for biobanks and bioresources. Procedures for collection, processing, storage and transportation technology criteria for either animal germplasm or for human genetic will be addressed by two different documents. In addition technical specifications for human biobanks and human bioresources in research and development will be addressed by a further document. The need to develop specific requirement for human resources derive from a series of ethical, legal and social issues that are peculiar to human biospecimens.

The release time of the WG2 ISO's norm (namely ISO 20387) is predicted to be: 8-12 months.

4.2. Scientific, Economic And Global Market Interest In Biobanking

Biobanks are not a new phenomenon, however, in the last decade there has been a global steep rate of increase that is contributing to the organizational diversity and growing complexity of the market for biobank services. In 2013, a U.S. national survey showed that over half of participating biobanks were established since 2001 [35], and tissue samples stored were expanding at a rate of approximately 20 million annually. In Europe, the inventory of major biobanks carried out during the preparatory phase of BBMRI, showed that 220 human biobanks hold more than 20 million biological samples [36].

The economic impact of biobanking is also growing, and even with a wide variation in estimates, all predictions report an increasing trend in most of sectors linked to bioresource use. The global biobanking market was valued at $186.3 billion in 2015. This market is expected to increase from $198.2 billion in 2016 to $240.2 billion in 2021 at a compound annual growth rate (CAGR) of 3.9% for 2016-2021 [37]. Interestingly, the private sector will experience the greatest increase. Although 5 years ago it represented the third sector in terms of revenue, it will became the first sector preceding both public and population segments. Furthermore, over 5years, population biobanks are also projected to grow from $57.8 billion in 2016 to $76.7 billion at a CAGR of 5.8% [37]. The availability of detailed requirements for the full range of activities and management procedures of biobanks will become of greater importance as biobanking and the market for biobank services are moving toward increased complexity, as well as a range of possible public-private partnerships, which are the true engines of biotechnological sample-based applications development. Expected medical and exploitable benefits include the discovery of new disease biomarkers and drug targets through large-scale and or novel molecular technologies, in addition to a generally enhanced understanding of disease mechanisms. As reported by BCC

Research [38], the global biomarkers market, which has grown to a CAGR of 19.7% from 2009 to 2014, showcases high growth potential also in the near future with an estimated CAGR of 12.4% from 2016 to 2021, to reach $71.03 billion by 2021 [38]. The percentage growth estimates may show some degree of heterogeneity, however all of them agree in confirming a growing trend for both individual disease markets and all health markets.

The growth of this market is driven by the rising demand for personalized medicine [39] and precision medicine [40] and finds fertile ground in the discovery technologies, government initiatives [41, 42], and grants for biomarker research.

Preserved tissues are an indispensable tool for the identification of molecular markers of response to specific innovative therapies, that may be already available or under development, and provide clinically useful information, such as, for example, the identification of disease risk markers for blood relatives.

In the area of biomarkers the "omics" technology segment holds the largest share of ~75% of the biomarker discovery market, primarily due to the increase in adoption of proteomics and genomics technologies globally. The main companies of the biotechnology sector, such as Roche Diagnostics Limited (Switzerland), Johnson & Johnson (U.S.), GlaxoSmithKline Plc. (U.K.), Siemens Healthcare (Germany), Abbott Laboratories Inc. (U.S.), GE Healthcare (U.K.), Affymetrix Inc. (U.S.), Epigenomics AG (Germany), Eisai Co. Ltd. (Japan), Bio-Rad Laboratories Inc. (U.S.), Eli Lilly and Company (U.S.), Merck & Co. (U.S.) are involved in this market and several model of partnerships have been implemented to ensure success in this sector [43].

Personalized medicine (treatment tailored to each individual patient) is also an engine for future pharmaceutical companies. So far, pharmaceutical products on the market target less than 500 human gene products. Even though not all of the 30.000 or so human protein coding genes will have products targetable for drug development, this suggests that there is an enormous untapped pool of human gene-based targets for therapeutic intervention.

The global market for drug discovery technologies and products reached $38.4 billion in 2011 and it is expected to expand from $41.4 billion in 2012 to $79.0 billion in 2017, a CAGR of 13.8% between 2012 and 2017. A further expanding sector is regenerative medicine, this is expected to grow to $4.6 billion by 2016 at a CAGR of 4.9%, and the Japanese Ministry of Economy, Trade and Industry in 2013 esteemed the global market in 2020 as approximately USD$20B [44].

4.3. Standard Setting Requires Solid Biobanking Knowledge

Although every effort has been made to maximize the comparability of biological samples-based study and applications across countries, caution must be used in comparing biobanking activities among countries when the data are obtained from studies with very different methodologies. Several factors such as differences in the definition of terms, whether or not all firms innovate, low response rates, whether or not results take account of non-respondents or are extrapolated to the total population, will all affect the comparability of achievements [45] and still hamper simple adoption of suitable models for public-private partnerships.

The basis for the solution for the task afforded by WG2 on biobanking is represented by solid scientific work that has been performed in recent years to improve both availability and access to qualifying samples. As mentioned before, P3G [24] made available a review of the most used guidelines and best practices for human samples, such as those produced by OECD [46] and NCI [47]. Many other initiatives contribute to a solid foundation for the work of theWG2. The CABRI (Common Access to Biological Resources and Information) working group was sponsored in 1996 by the European Commission and is a pioneering initiative aiming to provide a European catalogue of available bio-resources and quality guidelines [48].

Other early initiatives include StrainInfo which is a web- based search catalogue for 60 Bioresource research centers for microorganisms [49]. Microorganisms cover an important part of bioresources and their authentication, characterisation, stable storage and supply are a major contribution to the knowledge-based bioeconomy as their uses continue to expand, not just food and healthcare, but in almost all areas of industry and environmental maintenance [50]. The conservation and utilization of microorganisms and development of knowledge-based bioeconomy is the mission of EMbaRC [50], which aims to provide a one-stop access to the collections of EMbaRC and of other previous EU projects such as CABRI and EBRCN. Another initiative focused on microorganisms is the Microbial Resources Research Infrastructure (MIRRI), an ESFRI' roadmap research infrastructure which aims to integrate European microbiological resources centers and support R&D in the field of microbial-based biotechnology [51].

Reference documents for the WG2 in the field of Culture Collections of The World are those produced by the Federation of Culture Collections (WFCC) [52] which developed guidelines for the collection, authentication, maintenance and distribution of cultures of microorganisms and cultured cells, and the European Culture Collections' Organisation (ECCO) [53] which focus the activity in promoting collaboration and exchange of ideas on culture collections.

Biological resources such as plants and crop diversity are associated with the development of agriculture and agro-technology and are essential in the growth of human populations and continuous development of civilizations. Gene banks play a key role worldwide on long-term conservation, availability and use of animals and plants genetics resources. For plants genetics resources around 7.5 million accessions are held in the world by Gene bank (FAO 2013). Development of new methods as genetic association mapping or genomic selection, the important amount of data (passport data, phenotyping, genotyping...) that are generated implies strong collaboration between the diverse actors of resources genetic conservation and characterization and also appropriate informatics system, which are strongly hampered by the heterogeneity and non-comparability of knowledge and data.

4.4. Methodology

WG2 on biobanking is 'horizontal' WG and it is not concerned with to developing application-specific standards, except where it has identified a clear gap in standardization and a business demand, and/or there is no existing ISO committee or other established international standards-setting body applying their expertise to related standards development. Open discussion and, where possible, harmonization will be primary methodology used in order to bring together what has been proven and stood the test of time. The goal is to reach a consensus, avoiding duplication and conflicts. Thus, sectors already highly regulated as, for instance, some areas related to food production, agriculture or pharmaceuticals will be not addressed. The preferred methodology is collaboration. TC276 cooperates with ISO/CASCO, a committee which studies the means of assessing the conformity of products, processes, services and management systems to appropriate standards, and with ISO/REMCO a Committee on reference materials. Liaisons with other TC which are already addressing standardizations of sectors related to biotechnology applications have been established. Table **2** reports a list of the liaisons with a brief note on the main sector of collaboration with the WG2. In addition, collaborations are also in place with relevant and on-going international projects, as are initiatives to ensure that participants in specific sectors have the requisite standardization tools to support their activities and to provide outreach and enabling coordination of mutual activities. WG2 is also collaborating with other standards organizations (BBMRI-ERIC),EDQM (European directorate for the quality of medicines & healthcare), ICH (The International Conference on Harmonisation of Technical Requirements for Registration of Pharmaceuticals for Human Use), ISBER and the ESBB (European, Middle Eastern and African Society for Biopreservation and

Biobanking), to ensure that stakeholders have the requisite standardization tools to support their use of biotechnologies in new applications and markets. Collaborations will ensure efficient common practical approaches are implemented in compliance with international standards and national policies and regulations. Norms and/or guidelines will cover issues related to ethical aspects, accessibility of biological resources, organizational and managerial aspects, infrastructure and facilities, sample processing requirements (related to WG4 "Bioprocessing" output) and Sample Testing requirements (related to WG3 "Analytical Methods" output).

The WG2 deliverable(s) will take into account specificities of ISO 9001 requirements formulated/adapted and requirements not covered by ISO 9001 but related to human biobanks and biological resources. In addition to the guidelines and the documents cited above, the French standard, NF S 96-900 Quality of biological resource centres (BRC) and the British Biobank Quality Standard [54] are also considered. Furthermore, WG2' work will lead to the identification of possible gaps and fill them with appropriate specifications. Collection, processing, storage and transportation technology criteria for animal, germplasm samples and human genetic resources will be specifically addressed by additional documents.

Table 2. ISO/TC276 Liaison.

		WG2 Major Collaboration fields
ISO/TC 212	Clinical Laboratory testing and *in vitro* Diagnostic Test Systems	Laboratory medicine, *in vitro* diagnostic test systems, including analytical procedures, analytical performance, laboratory safety, reference systems and quality assurance
ISO/TC 34/SC 16	Horizontal Methods for Molecular Biomarker Analysis	Methods for nucleic acids and proteins analysis in foods, seeds and other propagates of food and feed crops
ISO/TC 48	Laboratory Equipment	Devices and apparatus for laboratory purposes, including materials of construction, performance, dimensions and testing
ISO/TC 61	Plastics	Biotechnology materials and products in the field of plastics
ISO/TC 147	Water Quality	Water quality,including definition of terms, sampling, measurement and reporting of water characteristics
ISO/TC 150/SC 7	Tissue- engineered Medical Products	Cell culture for self-replacement of tissues and organs; standards functional requirements both mechanical and biological for tissue- engineered products
ISO/TC 184	Automation Systems and Integration	Interface and integrate standardization in the field of automation systems, such as information systems, robotics for fixed and mobile robots automation and control software and integration technologies

(Table 2) contd.....

		WG2 Major Collaboration fields
ISO/TC 194/SC1	Tissue Product Safety	Biocompatibility, biological evaluation and safety of animal tissues and their derivatives utilized in the manufacture of medical devices
ISO/TC 215	Health Information	Health informatics to facilitate the creation, interchanges and use of health-related data, information, and knowledge to support and enable all aspects of the health system
CEN/TC 140	*In- vitro* Diagnostic Medical Devices	*In vitro* diagnostic medical devices, such as reagents, kits, instruments, apparatus, equipment, or system, which are used for the examination of specimens, including blood and tissue donations derived from the human
CEN/TC 233	Biotechnology	Food, pharmaceuticals and agriculture biotechnology
CEN/TC275/WG1	Genetically Modified Foodstuffs	Genetically modified organism sand food:food ingredients produced from, but not containing, genetically modified organisms
CEN/TC 316	Medical Products Utilizing Cells, Tissues and/or their Derivatives	Medical products manufactured utilizing animal and/or human tissues, cells and/or their derivatives
CEN/TC 411	Bio-Based Products	Consistent terminology, sampling, certification tools, bio-based content, application of and correlation towards life cycle analysis, sustainability criteria for biomass used and for final products

CONCLUDING REMARKS

Efforts made so far in all aspects of biobanking to facilitate public-private relationships are impressive, however, they have not been able to offer to the users "one-stop shopping" bioresources, which is a pivotal request of private sectors [55]. In general terms, the ISO standard for research biobanking will be the result of international, expert consensus and therefore offer the benefit of global management experience and good practice. To improve access to qualifying samples will require more efficient use of resources, improved risk management, and an increase in trust between any type of stakeholders (either provider/recipient or funders) and clients/citizens. The ISO norm can be applied to any organization, large or small, whatever the product or service and regardless of the sector of activity, and facilitate better science, excellent and innovative medicine. The biobanking norm will provide simply and unequivocally expressed requirements, specifications, guidelines or characteristics can be used consistently to ensure that materials, products, processes and services are *fit for their purpose*. In other words, the ISO biobanking standard will be the standardized guidance for implementation of QMS in biobanking, providing an *ad hoc* certification system with global reach. It can be envisaged as a large umbrella that covers all processes in a biobank, from collection to storing, including disposal, data management, safeguarding, distribution and transportation for any type of biological samples. The scope goes beyond methodological operating procedures to include ethical and regulatory issues as well as data annotations related to samples.

The certification of the biobank will be a way to communicate that it has the ability to ensure the appropriate quality in the collection, the preservation and the distribution of biological materials and of the services offered. It will certify that the biobank operates according to worldwide recognized guiding principles and operating procedures which guarantee the quality of biobanking activities and improve the social trust. This system will allow information to be effectively exchanged by the parties/partners, allowing knowledge to be disseminated reliably in a defined language. It will generate trust leading to an optimization of collaboration/contracts and ultimately to reduction of time and costs, which in turn, in a virtuous cycle, will incentivize the adoption of quality principles. Outputs from the standardization in association with reliable the certification system of MSS will facilitate biotechnological development, support national and international competitiveness, contribute to the predictability of the regulatory environment, support the exchange of goods and services through the elimination of technical barriers, and support market access.

CONFLICT OF INTEREST

The authors confirm that they have no conflict of interest to declare for this publication.

ACKNOWLEDGEMENT

We are grateful to the Ministry of Health and to the Ministry of Education, University and Research for the support given to the ISS to sustain work on biobanking. We are thankful to Prof. Kathleen M. Botham for her helpful advice during the review process and English revision of the manuscript.

REFERENCES

[1]   Deming WE, Ed. The New Economics for Industry, Government, and Education. Boston, Ma: MIT Press 1993; p. 132.

[2]   Statistical Method From the Viewpoint of Quality Control US Department of Agriculture. Reprinted by Dover 1939; p. 45.

[3]   Martínez-Lorente AR, Dewhurst FD, Barrie G. Total Quality Management: Origins and Evolution of the Term. TQM Mag 1998; 10: 378-86.
[http://dx.doi.org/10.1108/09544789810231261]

[4]   Grizzle WE, Gunter EW, Sexton KC, Bell WC. Quality management of biorepositories. Biopreserv Biobank 2015; 13(3): 183-94.
[http://dx.doi.org/10.1089/bio.2014.0105] [PMID: 26035008]

[5]   Simeon-Dubach D, Watson P. Biobanking 3.0: evidence based and customer focused biobanking. Clin

Biochem 2014; 47(4-5): 300-8.
[http://dx.doi.org/10.1016/j.clinbiochem.2013.12.018] [PMID: 24406300]

[6]   Vaught J, Kelly A, Hewitt R. A review of international biobanks and networks: success factors and key benchmarks. Biopreserv Biobank 2009; 7(3): 143-50.
[http://dx.doi.org/10.1089/bio.2010.0003] [PMID: 24835880]

[7]   Asian Consortium for the Conservation and Sustainable Utilization of Microbial Resources: http://www.acm-mrc.asia

[8]   China National Gene Bank: http://www.nationalgenebank.org/en/

[9]   Chen H, Pang T. A call for global governance of biobanks. Bull World Health Organ 2015; 93(2): 113-7.
[http://dx.doi.org/10.2471/BLT.14.138420] [PMID: 25883404]

[10]   Fraunhofer IB. Case Study on the Economic Impact of Biobanks Illustrated by EuroCryo Saar 2009. Available from: http://www.tissuebank.it/publicazioni/docUfficiale/DocumentazioneScientifica/ BBMRI-Fraunhofer-Case-Study-final.pdf/

[11]   BBMRI: an evaluation strategy for socio-economic impact assessment 2013. Available from http://www.technopolis-group.com/resources/downloads/life_sciences/1093_BBMRIfinalreport_1009 21.pdf

[12]   Cambon-Thomsen A. The social and ethical issues of post-genomic human biobanks. Nat Rev Genet 2004; 5(11): 866-73.
[http://dx.doi.org/10.1038/nrg1473] [PMID: 15520796]

[13]   Lenk C. Donors and Users of Human tissues for research purpose from Trust in Biobanking: Trust in Biobanking: Dealing with Ethical, Legal and Social Issues in an Emerging Field of Biotechnology. In: Science S, Media B, Eds. Peter Dabrock, JochenTaupitz, Jens Ried. 2012; pp. 83-97.

[14]   Bromley RL. Financial stability in biobanking: unique challenges for disease-focused foundations and patient advocacy organizations. Biopreserv Biobank 2014; 12(5): 294-9.
[http://dx.doi.org/10.1089/bio.2014.0053] [PMID: 25313427]

[15]   Rudan I, Marušić A, Campbell H. Developing biobanks in developing countries. J Glob Health 2011; 1(1): 2-4.
[PMID: 23198094]

[16]   Emerson CI, Singer PA, Upshur RE. Access and use of human tissues from the developing world: ethical challenges and a way forward using a tissue trust. BMC Med Ethics 2011; 12: 2-5.
[http://dx.doi.org/10.1186/1472-6939-12-2] [PMID: 21266076]

[17]   Morris K. Revising the Declaration of Helsinki. Lancet 2013; 381(9881): 1889-90.
[http://dx.doi.org/10.1016/S0140-6736(13)60951-4] [PMID: 23734387]

[18]   Framework for Responsible Sharing of Genomic and Health-Related Data. Toronto: The Global Alliance for Genomics and Health 2014. Available from: http://genomicsandhealth.org/ files/public/FrameworkforResponsibleSharingofGenomicandHealth- RelatedDataVersion2010September2014.pdf

[19]   Calzolari A, Valerio A, Capone F, *et al.* The European Research Infrastructures of the ESFRI Roadmap in Biological and Medical Sciences: status and perspectives. Ann Ist Super Sanita 2014; 50(2): 178-85.
[PMID: 24968918]

[20]   Biobanking and Biomolecular Resources Research Infrastructure: http://www.p3g.org/

[21]   Public Population Project in Genomics and Society: http://www.p3g.org

[22]   International Society for Biological and Environmental Repositories: http://www.isber.org/

[23]   International Agency for Research on Cancer: http://ibb.iarc.fr/

[24]   P3G Montreal: Public Population Project in Genomics and Society 2014. Available from: http://www.p3g.org/system/files/biobank_toolkit_documents/Comparison%20Chart%20Guidelines_20 08-05-14-update%202009-08-03_0.pdf

[25]   Chen H. A Case Study of China KadoorieBiobank. Sci Technol Soc 2013; 18: 321-38.
[http://dx.doi.org/10.1177/0971721813498497]

[26]   Ndebele P, Musesengwa R. Will developing countries benefit from their participation in genetics research? Malawi Med J 2008; 20(2): 67-9.
[http://dx.doi.org/10.4314/mmj.v20i2.10960] [PMID: 19537436]

[27]   Puchois P. Finding ways to improve the use of biobanks. Nat Med 2013; 19(7): 814-5.
[http://dx.doi.org/10.1038/nm.3257] [PMID: 23836219]

[28]   ISO/TC 276 Biotechnology: Available from: http://www.iso.org/ iso/home/standards_development/ list_of_iso_technical_committees/iso_technical_committee.htm?commid=4514241

[29]   International Accreditation Forum: htpp://www.iaf.nu

[30]   European Accreditation: http://www.european-accreditation.org/ea-members

[31]   Brigitte van Beuzekom B, Arundel A. OECD Biotechnology statistics 2006. Available from: http://www.oecd.org/science/inno/36760212.pdf

[32]   The Bioeconomy to 2030: Designing a policy agenda. OECD 2009. Available from: http://www.oecd.org/futures/long-termtechnologicalsocietalchallenges/42837897.pdf

[33]   JRC reference report, Consequences, Opportunities and Challenges of Biotechnology for Europe 2007. Available from http://ipts.jrc.ec.europa.eu/publications/pub.cfm?id=1470

[34]   Bravo E. Biotecnologie: Nuove risposte ai problemi esistenti e alle sfide future. U&C 2015; 7: 29-30.

[35]   Henderson GE, Cadigan RJ, Edwards TP, *et al.* Characterizing biobank organizations in the U.S: results from a national survey. Genome Med 2013; 5(1): 3.
[http://dx.doi.org/10.1186/gm407] [PMID: 23351549]

[36]   Wichmann HE, Kuhn KA, Waldenberger M, *et al.* Comprehensive catalog of European biobanks. Nat Biotechnol 2011; 29(9): 795-7.
[http://dx.doi.org/10.1038/nbt.1958] [PMID: 21904320]

[37]   Biobanking: Technologies and Global Markets: http://www.bccresearch.com/market-research/ biotechnology/biobanking-technologies-markets-report-bio084b.html

[38]   BCC   Research:
http://www.marketsandmarkets.com/Market-Reports/top-10-bioprocess-technology-market-30722776. html

[39]   Keeling P, Roth M, Zietlow T. The economics of personalized medicine: commercialization as a driver of return on investment. N Biotechnol 2012; 29(6): 720-31.
[http://dx.doi.org/10.1016/j.nbt.2012.06.001] [PMID: 22713855]

[40]   Toward Precision Medicine: Building a Knowledge Network for Biomedical Research and a New Taxonomy of Disease Washington (DC). US: National Academies Press 2011.

[41]   Collins FS, Varmus H. A new initiative on precision medicine. N Engl J Med 2015; 372(9): 793-5.
[http://dx.doi.org/10.1056/NEJMp1500523] [PMID: 25635347]

[42]   Personalised medicine in Europe: a great challenge for improving patient care 2013. Available from: http://epthinktank.eu/

[43]   Biomarkers Market Analysis and Reports-USA Conference Series - Biomarkers 2017 2017. Available from: http://market-analysis.conferenceseries.com/biomarkers-market-reports

[44]   Announcement of the Final Report Compiled by the Study Group on Commercialization and Industrialization of Regenerative Available from: http://www.meti.go.jp/english/press/2013/

0222_03.html

[45]   M45] Economic, Environmental and Social Statistics 2014. Available from http://www.oecd-ilibrary.org/sites/factbook-2014-en/index.html

[46]   OECD Best practise guidelines 2007 Available from http://www.oecd.org/sti/biotech/38777417.pdf

[47]   NCI Best Practices for Biospecimen Resources 2011. Available from https://biospecimens.cancer.gov/bestpractices/2011-ncibestpractices.pdf

[48]   Common Access to Biological Resources and Information: http://www.cabri.org/guidelines.html

[49]   World Data Center for Microorganism: http://www.wfcc.info/ccinfo/collection/by_region/Asia/

[50]   European Consortium of Microbial Resources Centres: http://www.embarc.eu/

[51]   Microbial Resources Research Infrastructure: http://www.mirri.org/home.html

[52]   Federation of Culture Collections: http://www.wfcc.info/

[53]   European Culture Collections' Organisation: https://www.eccosite.org/

[54]   Biobank-quality-standard: Available from: http://ccb.ncri.org.uk/wp-content/uploads/2014/03/Biobank-quality-standard-Version-1.pdf

[55]   Madore SJ. Biobanking for genomics-based translational medicine. In: Kumar D, Eng C, Eds. Genomic Medicine- Principles and Practice. 2014; pp. 235-41.

CHAPTER 4

Quality Criteria in Oncology: Lessons learned from the B4MED Biobank

Giancarlo Pruneri[1,2] and **Giuseppina Bonizzi**[3,*]

[1] Director, Biobank for Translational Medicine Unit, European Institute of Oncology, Milan

[2] Associate Professor in Pathology, University of Milan, School of Medicine

[3] Executive coordinator of Biobank for Translational Medicine Unit, European Oncology Institute (IEO), Milan, Italy

Abstract: Since the beginning, the scientific research was an integral part of the mission of the European Oncology Institute (IEO). Its position is at the intersection between Surgical Units, the Department of Pathology and Research Units. This organization makes the IEO Biobank for Translational Medicine (B4MED) a critical resource that reflects the mission of IEO to perform "Research for Care".

The B4MED collects, catalogues and stores biological samples that are non-essential for diagnostic purposes from patients who provide informed consent for the use of their tissues for research purposes. A direct pipeline with the operating theatres for the collection of tissue samples ensures negligible sample degradation. Surgically-excised pathological and non-pathological tissue samples, plasma/serum, total blood, DNA and RNA are collected and stored according to specific protocols and standard operating procedures. All biobanked samples are managed and tracked through a software package that is fully integrated with the hospital medical records database, pathology database and central registry of patient demographic information. This ensures that each sample is linked to a full complement of anonymous or anonymized (according to patient choice) patient information that is accessible solely by authorized Biobank personnel.

The high quality biospecimens collected by the B4MED are used for biomarker and drug discovery experiments, both for basic research and for clinical research, with the ultimate aim of providing excellence in patient care through excellence in research.

Keywords: B4MED IEOBiobank for Translational Medicine Unit, Handling, Participation Pact, Pathological and non pathological, Sample collection, Storage and news approach for the pathologist work, Trust-based consent.

---

* **Corresponding author Giuseppina Bonizzi:** Executive coordinator of Biobank for Translational Medicine Unit, European Oncology Institute (IEO), Milan, Italy; Tel: +393493203787; Email: giuseppina.bonizzi@ieo.it

Elena Salvaterra and Julie Corfield (Eds.)
All rights reserved-© 2017 Bentham Science Publishers

INTRODUCTION

In the last two decades, progress in biomedical disciplines has made fundamental steps towards the identification of pathogenic processes, genetic disorders, specific pathways and molecular targets in inflammatory and oncologic diseases, that has open up the new era of targeted personalized medicine [1, 2].

These achievements have been possible also thanks to the implementation of biobanks which are collections of different human biological samples organized following strict ethical, statistical and biological procedures [3, 4].

In this chapter we will discuss important requirements of a modern biobank by describing the organization and quality control criteria implemented from the tissue bank of the European Oncology Institute (IEO) based in Milan, Italy (*i.e.* Biobank for Translational Medicine Unit).

This biobank collects catalogues and stores biological samples (namely, surgically excised tissue samples non-essential for diagnosis, plasma/serum, total blood, DNA and RNA) donated from patients who provided informed consent for the storage and use of their tissues and cells for research purposes. In particular we will report the comprehensive pipeline that links in traceable and semi-automatic way the various phases of the process that include: a) the collection of a new form of trust-based consent (the so-called Participation Pact), b) the collection and processing of tissue samples, cells, plasma, serum, total blood, DNA and RNA that are subsequently stored according to specific protocols and standard operating procedures (SOPs).

Additionally, primary cell cultures, stem cell preparations, and tissues from animals xenotransplanted with tumors are stored in our facility, by providing researchers and physicians with valuable biomaterial for research purposes.

The Participation Pact A New Form Of Trust-Based Consent

The first issue to be considered in relation to the collection and storage of human biological specimens is about the ethical requirements to be met for legitimate use of samples and it refers to the informed consent of subjects participating in research using their biological materials and or associated data.

With regard to this issue, only biological specimens deriving from patients who have signed a specially designed informed consent for research purposes are accepted to be banked in our facility [5, 6].

Accordingly a new form of trust-based consent for research biobanks has been specifically implemented [7]. The trust-based consent, the so-called Participation

Pact(P-P), has two fundamental features.

Firstly, it defines a new form of relationship between researchers and participants based on mutual trust. In this way, the two parties are bound by a pact, which prevents the relationship from being unbalanced and forces both parties to respect the agreement they have forged [7].

Secondly, participation in research is completely transformed. Unlike previous models that attempted to impose on participants a robust duty to participate in research [7], a pact-based relationship instead provides participants with a strong incentive to do so, as they are motivated by an act of solidarity where reciprocity, trust and the belief that science is an ethical enterprise play mutual supportive roles [7].

With the P-P, patients can choose whether or not to donate samples for research purposes and are offered the choice of samples being held either anonymously or being anonymized with a specific encryption that avoids to retrieve patient identity compliant with privacy National laws [7].

Furthermore, audio-visual material has been prepared to explain the main features of the P-P and to help patients make fully informed decisions to participate or not to our research programs by donating biological samples. To ensure maximum compliance, trained Biobank research nurses are always on hand to explain to patients the impact and implications of their decision [7].

Collection and Management of Data Relating to Samples

All biobanked samples are managed and tracked through a software package that is fully integrated with the hospital medical records database and pathology database. This is essential in order to timely manage high quality clinical data linked to all biospecimens collected by the Biobank for Translational Medicine Unit.

These specimens are then used for biomarker and drug discovery experiments, both for basic research and for translational research projects (*e.g.* the development of personalized therapies), with the ultimate aim of providing excellence in patient care through excellence in research.

This was also achieved by the integration of its activity with the Department of Pathology, which ensures the continued and centralized supervision of a dedicated pathologist in the processing of biomaterials in an *ad hoc* structured core facility. Specimen collection can be institutional or linked to a specific project driven by a researcher.

In both the cases the approval by Technical and Scientific Committee of IEO is necessary to collect and use the stored samples. As example, the samples collected in our facility come from the Divisions of breast, thoracic, gynecology and urology. In addition to tumoral and non-tumoral tissue, we also collect blood, serum and plasma. Furthermore depending on the requirements of each specific project our Biobank is also equipped with specific procedures for the collection of biopsies, feces, urine, ascetic fluid and saliva. In selected cases, and only for patients that signed an additional specific consent for the study, DNA, RNA, primary cell cultures, stem cell preparations, and tissues from animals xenotransplanted with tumors derived from collected samples are stored in our facility.

Sample Collection, Handling, and Storage

Sample collection from surgical specimens for biobanking must be an integral part of clinical practice. At the moment, we collect all biological samples related to the divisions of breast, thoracic, gynecology and urology. For each patient we collect in addition to the normal and pathological tissue, blood, serum and plasma.

Moreover we collect fresh samples for xenotrasplantation, cell culture, DNA or RNA extraction. While frozen tissue is the gold standard, all sample types should be collected where possible. Multiple samples must also be collected.

For each tumour type, a ranking order should be established. This would indicate which type of sample processing should be available for all cases, and which types of processing should be carried out if sufficient material were available.

Pilot studies/feasibility should be carried out around specific disease areas/sample types in order to ensure that the appropriate and practical standards are applied. The relevant laboratory should perform sample processing in order to ensure that only the material that has been requested by the researcher is actually released, thus avoiding the unnecessary waste of valuable material.

The large numbers of samples available for collaborations will create much greater potential for translational research projects and will facilitate clinical trials.

If samples from different collection sites, or indeed from the same site, are to be comparable, they must be collected in a standardized way, and they must be processed and stored according to the same protocols as far as possible.

All assessments of quality should be adequately recorded both in relation to the methods employed and the results obtained. The Quality Control (QC) for sample collection, processing and annotation must be standardized.

The QC should include recording the time from actual cancer resection to the freezing of samples in the biobank.

Appropriate QC such as Haematoxylin and Eosin (H&E) staining of sections and/or immunostaining must be performed for each specimen. Where possible, a H&E section should be taken from an adjacent (paraffin) block, to confirm that a lesion is present and to determine what percentage of the sample it accounts for.

DNA and RNA integrity should be tested on a defined percentage of samples. A pathologist must review all patient tissue specimens to determine what material can be made available for research and the optimal samples and number of aliquots to be taken. Bloods and other body fluids not required for diagnosis can be collected in accordance with approved protocols and do not require pathologic review but quality control.

Stored biomaterials include surgically removed tissue specimens and blood samples or other biological fluid samples, such as urine, saliva, *etc.*

Biomaterials are either stored in special cryopreservation systems including freezers at –80°C or liquid nitrogen tanks.

Tissues are frozen following two different methods, one envisaging the use of cryovials and one envisaging the use of cryomolds and OCT. Multiple samples, when it is possible, are made with pathological, and non pathological, using both methods.

Tissues are frozen by immersion in pre-cooled isopentane (2-methyl butane) and stored in freezers at –80°C and in liquid nitrogen tanks. All biomaterials are labeled with a barcode (2D), univocal and secret that enable to handle them while maintaining the patient anonymity when required.

Collection And Management of Data Related to Samples

Appropriate software that is connected with the hospital medical record database and the pathology database collects data concerning the specimens stored in the IEO biobank. The software is specifically designed to address the unique challenges of specimen collection, tracking, and storage for pharmaceutical discovery and clinical operations, academic and biosciences, research centers, medical institutions and contract research organizations (CROs).

The information is correlated to clinical, pathological and genetic data of the patient, mainly processed, in electronic manner, by legacy systems of the

Operative Unit of Pathological Anatomy, clinical record and personal data of the IEO. Other clinical information derived from the different database, present in the different department of the hospital and from the Tumor Registry.

Biosafety

The handling of human tissues implies the risk of possible exposure to pathogens. The presence of infectious agents in stored biomaterials cannot actually be excluded. In order to minimize these risks, the personnel handling the material stored in biobank must consider all specimens as potentially infectious.

Moreover, before collection of the samples we always look for the risk of infection. All the sample that are risk infection (positive for HIV, HCV, e HBV) are discarded, even if the patient have signed the Participation Agreement.

Patient's Enrolment

The patients come enrolled on the basis of the selection criteria, specific for each disease. The only situation that we usually exclude is the risk infectious known as previously reported.

Nurses who have followed a specific training to learn the way to explain the different topics included collect the consent.

The somministration may be made during pre-hospitalization, before or doing an exam or during hospitalization.

Selection criteria of biological samples from patients of surgery are different in function of the treated disease. An example of used criteria is reported as follows:

SELECTION CRITERIA OF BIOLOGICAL SAMPLES FROM ABDOMINOPELVIC

Eligibility criteria:

• Patients operated for emicolectomie.

SELECTION CRITERIA OF BIOLOGICAL SAMPLES FROM PATIENTS OF PLASTIC SURGERY

Eligibility criteria Champions Anatomical:

• Patients operated for mastectomies reductive
    Exclusion criteria:
• Patients who do not are included in the eligibility criteria.

SELECTION CRITERIA OF BIOLOGICAL SAMPLES FROM PATIENTS OF PREVENTIVE GYNECOLOGY

Eligibility criteria:

- Patients operated for gynecological diseases not included in the categories described in the exclusion criteria;
- Patients with recurrent gynecologic cancers operated as per protocol;
- Patients with previous treatments (chemotherapy or radiotherapy).
    Exclusion criteria Champions Anatomical:
- Patients who are at genetic risk (familiar for ovarian cancer and/or breast) and BRCA1/2 changed;
- Patients with a history Breast cancer;
- Patients where the ovarian cancer and 'to be considered as metastasis from another tumor (*e.g.* Colon, *etc.*);
    Eligibility criteria of Biological Fluids:
- Subjects without gynecological diseases known, who have filled out the medical history questionnaire;
- Subjects relating to the IEO for screening for gynecological diseases (*e.g.* Pap-test);
- Patients undergoing ovarectomyprophylactic or hysterectomies (both pre-operative and post-operative);
- Patients who are at genetic risk (familiar for ovarian cancer and/or breast) and BRCA1/2 changed;
- All patients operated for gynecological pathologies that meet the eligibility criteria Champions Anatomical.
    Exclusion criteria of Biological Fluids:
- Patients with a history Breast cancer (except for Preventive Gynecology);
- Patients where the ovarian cancer and 'to be considered as metastasis from another tumor (*e.g.* Colon, *etc.*);

SELECTION CRITERIA FOR THE LEVY OF BLOOD AND BIOLOGICAL SAMPLES FROM PATIENTS OF SENOLOGY

Eligibility criteria Champions Anatomical:
  ○ Patients diagnosed with breast cancer;
  ○ Patients with suspected breast cancer;
  ○ Patients BRCA1/2 changed;
  ○ Controlateral cancer.
Eligibility criteria of Biological Fluids:
  ○ Patients in the course of investigations (second level of screening);
Follow Up • Patients diagnosed with breast cancer;
  ○ Subjects relating to the IEO for mammograms and ultrasounds of first

access;
○ Patients BRCA1/2 changed;
○ All patients diagnosed with breast cancer.

Exclusion criteria Champions Anatomical and Organic Liquids:
○ Tumors with diameters of less than 0.5 centimeters (pT1a) are not collected (but we collected only the blood and serum sample;
○ Previous cancer (excluding Paget's disease, basal cell carcinoma and CIN);
○ Prior treatment (CT and/or RT);
○ Recurrence of breast cancer;
○ Metastatic carcinoma;
○ Benign;
○ Tumors *in situ* (DIN)

SELECTION CRITERIA OF BIOLOGICAL SAMPLES FROM PATIENTS OF THORACIC SURGERY

Eligibility criteria Champions Anatomical:
○ All patients operated on for lung cancer;
○ All types of N2 lung cancers;
○ Patients with previous chemotherapy treatments (particularly for lung tumors of type N2);
○ Patients with lung cancer belonging to Education COSMOS1 and COSMOS2 and their follow-up that comply with the protocol.

Eligibility criteria of Biological Fluids:
○ All patients operated on for lung cancer;
○ All patients in the study and COSMOS1 COSMOS2 that respect the protocol;
○ All patients in follow-up and that 'something stored in the Biobank.

Exclusion criteria Champions Anatomical and Organic Liquids:
○ Patients where the lung cancer and 'to be considered as metastasis of another tumor.

SELECTION CRITERIA OF BIOLOGICAL SAMPLES FROM PATIENTS UROLOGY

Eligibility criteria Champions Anatomical:
○ Patients with prostate cancer undergoing robotic prostatectomy prior multi-parametric MRI as per protocol;
○ Patients with advanced bladder cancer undergoing radical cystoprosta-tectomy as per protocol.

Exclusion criteria Champions Anatomical:
○ Prior treatment (CT and/or RT);
○ Recurrent

Sampling Protocols for Specific Organs: Some Examples

Based on these criteria, we wrote in detail with the help of pathologists the sampling protocol specific for thoracic, urology and gynecology department.

Here are some examples of considerable innovation of two sampling as:

Sampling Protocol for Lung Cancer Tissue Bank for Patients Study Enrolled Cosmos

For tumors larger than 1 cm sampling is done in accordance with the criteria for eligibility 'of the tissue bank.

For tumors smaller than one cm without preoperative diagnosis with the procedure involves the following steps:

1. Surgical resection of the nodule (wedge or segmentectomy).
2. Opening of the workpiece by the surgeon, taking care to divide the nodule into two halves in the operating room and macroscopic evaluation of the lesion.
3. In case of suspicion for inflammatory lesion in the operating room performing pad on nodule and the taking of samples of a few mm for bacterial culture to maintain a sterile field.
4. Enter the piece open (any signaling point with the area of greatest uptake in case of injury inconspicuous but localized with *technetium*).
5. Removal of one half of the cross section of tumor nodule of approximately 1 mm thickness for extemporaneous histological examination by the pathologist for diagnosis.
6. Once the diagnosis sampling of tumor tissue and healthy that will be made by the pathologist even if the lump is less than cm (the pathologist will make the diagnosis and to have enough material to the final).
7. Only in case of doubtful histology and of little material in the opinion of the pathologist will be able to use the frozen blocks extemporaneous examination for the tissue bank.

For tumors smaller than one cm but with preoperative diagnosis of tumour sampling to the bank of the fabric is performed by the pathologist reference to protocol of the bank of the fabric even if the nodule appears smaller than the cm and at the discretion of the pathologist.

For nodules of the patients included in the randomized protocol of limited resections pathologist (preferably with the surgeon) will measure both the larger diameter of the nodule that the distance from the margins prior to sampling for extemporaneous.

Prostate

Make withdrawals of fresh tissue in the prostate is a complex maneuver, difficult to perform due to the shape of the organ itself, for the sampling procedure pathological (usually done after fixation in neutral buffered formalin) useful for the diagnosis and the implications clinical and therapeutic follow.

Anatomically, the prostate is in fact contained in a capsule that incorporates the neurovascular bundles. The integrity of the capsule is a prerequisite for proper evaluation of the histopathological radical surgery. In addition, the macroscopic evaluation of the presence or absence of neoplastic lesions is often ineffective, since in most cases, the prostate cancer is not organized spatially to form lesions macroscopically appreciable, but rather winds between the non-neoplastic tissue structures. In other words, unlike other organs, for which the cutting, the visualization and the collection of tissue in fresh, whether it be neoplastic, be it non-neoplastic, are free from difficulties and complications, for prostate, it is necessary to in place a series of measures, beginning with the experience and expertise of the medical pathologist.

In order to properly assess the radical surgery, the entire outer surface of the bowel is marked with ink or special acrylic paints of different colors to indicate the laterality and other elements useful for diagnosis (vascular and nervous, burglary capsular, previous biopsies examined with intraoperative histological examination).

Based on the outcome of the examination inspection and palpation, assisted, where available, the mapping obtained by multi-parametric MRI, the pathologist selects areas to be sampled and the methods of cutting organ.

Prostatectomy

Prostatectomy can be performed in two steps:

- CLEAN CUT ONE, transverse to the major axis of the organ, from the rear face, in correspondence of any lump found or suspected areas reported by multi-parametric MRI, without completing the cut. You obtain two halves held together by fibro-muscular of the front area, each of which offers to consider a portion of tissue protruding over the cutting surfaces. By making a further cut parallel to that previously made and still without affecting the capsule, you can take the share of excess tissue. In cases where there is an appreciable proportion of excess tissue, it can affect the surface obtained by cutting prostate, taking away small fragment of parallelepiped shape, without affecting the capsule.

The pathologist indicates properly the seat of the levy, so that we can confirm histologically the nature of the same, whether neoplastic or non-neoplastic. The conclusion of the budget provides for the closure of two halves with appropriate restraints, making sure that the edges are aligned and that the pseudo capsule has not been reversed, before storing the bowels in a container with adequate amount of formalin.

- By serial cuts parallel to each other and transverse axis of the prostate, after removing the apex and the base of the prostate. The cuts are those that are performed normally on tissue fixed in formalin, according to sampling protocols. Sections of variable thickness, from 3 to 5 mm, are obtained and these sections allow an easier inspection and palpation aimed at identifying suspicious areas and suggestive of malignancy.

In some cases, especially when the shape of the organ is irregular, you can use a suitable tool (Prost-cut) provided with slits through which lead the blade to obtain sections of regular and uniform thickness. Even with this technique, each section has to consider a share of parenchyma which protrudes over the cutting surfaces, usable for cultures or tissue to be frozen, in the manner already described, using the mapping organ reproduced by the RMN multi-parametric.

Alternatively, if no appreciably adequate portion of tissue can be taken, it may affect the cut surface, removing a fragment of healthy tissue, preserving the capsule, as already described. The locations of the levy are marked for histological confirmation of cancer or benign. The conclusion of the maneuver provides, in this case, the drafting of the sections and their immobilization with suitable supports, on sheets of polystyrene or crushed directly in macrobius-cassettes in order to avoid changes in the shape and thickness, due to the contractions of the fibromuscular parenchyma of the prostate. Particular attention is paid to the pseudo-capsule so that it is flat all around the tissue sections. Finally, everything together at the apex, the base and the seminal vesicles, are placed in a container with adequate amount of formalin.

Cystoprostatectomy

In the case of cystoprostatectomy (in patients suffering from bladder cancer) sampling of the prostate will take place with one of the methods described above, taking care to leave intact the portion of the bladder neck necessary for the "closing" of the bladder that will be sampled, after fixation which also involves the distension of the organ prior insufflation of formalin, such as by standard procedures.

Ovary

The pathologist will use just tissues removed during surgery for sampling fragments to be allocated to this study. The sample of neoplastic tissue frankly, where the tumor component typically occupies a large part of the lesion, is not particularly difficult. Even the removal of ascites, which will be performed intraoperatively, is now part of routine operations. Conversely, special attention will be devoted to sampling ovarian and tubal tissue macroscopically not pathological.

As regards the ovary, the primary cell cultures will be derived from epithelium surface [8], or the monolayer of mesothelial cells that lines the organ. Consequently, the sampling will be carried out *via* dissection sagittal ovary, so as to obtain an adequate amount of cortical tissue. In particular, it will proceed to dissection of the outermost portion of the ovarian cortex with a depth of 2-3 mm for an extension of about 1-2 cm^2.

In case of withdrawal of tube not pathological, on the assumption that high-grade tumors are derived primarily from the fimbriae, the sampling will be carried out through the cut of about 1/10 of the pavilion with the fimbriae distal previously "open". Where possible, the sampling also expect fragments of dell' endosalpinx of the most proximal segment of the tube (infundibulum), the purpose of comparing the presence and the properties of stem cells [8] derived from the two different portions tubal

CONCLUSION

The collection and storage of bio-material strictly annotated with related clinical data provides a rich resource for the scientific community and represent the bridge for translational research, resulting in improvements in health and welfare of people. To this end, biobanks are increasingly recognized as critical resources to support research in a timely way, especially now that personalized medicine has increasing importance both for predictive and preventive medicine.

Regarding cancer biobanks, a valuable source of tissues/organs for research are both quality and accessibility of samples, and the extent of information stored together with tissues. To this end it is of fundamental importance, the sampling of the surgical specimen by the pathologist, so that it is carried out ensuring a correct diagnosis on the one hand and on the other the possibility of doing research with adequate tissue preparations.

In our biobank, specific operational procedures are well settled and respected, thus using standardized procedures complying with ISO 9001 certification in the context of biobanks for research.

CONFLICT OF INTEREST

The authors confirm that they have no conflict of interest to declare for this publication.

ACKNOWLEDGEMENT

The authors wish to acknowledge Maria Capra and Fulvia Fusar for their role in data management, and Giulio Taliento, Andrea Uggetti, Maria Lucia Longo and Cristina Cassi for all biobanking work.

REFERENCES

[1]   Gainer VS CA, Castro VM, Duey S, *et al.* The Biobank Portal for Partners Personalized Medicine: A Query Tool for Working with Consented Biobank Samples, Genotypes, and Phenotypes Using i2b2. J Pers Med 2016 Feb 26; 6(1): 11.

[2]   Judita Kinkorová. Biobanks in the era of personalized medicine: objectives, challenges, and innovation: Overview. EPMA J 2016 Feb 22; 7: 4.

[3]   Riegman PH MM, Betsou F, de Blasio P, Geary P. Marble Arch International Working Group on Biobanking for Biomedical Research., Biobanking for better healthcare. Mol Oncol 2008 Jul 30; Oct; 2 (3): 213-2.

[4]   Jonas Astrin SB, Thomas J, Barr EB, *et al.* Best Practices for Repositories Collection, Storage, Retrieval, and Distribution of Biological Materials for Research. Biopreserv Biobank 2012; 10(2): 79-161.

[5]   Hoeyer K. The Ethics of Research Biobanking: A Critical Review of the Literature. Biotechnol Genet Eng Rev 2008; 25: 429-52.
[http://dx.doi.org/10.5661/bger-25-429] [PMID: 21412365]

[6]   Cervo S, RJ, Talamini R, Perin T, Canzonieri V, De Paoli P, Steffan A. An effective multisource informed consent procedure for research and clinical practice: an observational study of patient understanding and awareness of their roles as research stakeholders in a cancer biobank. BMC Med Ethics 2013; 14: 30.
[http://dx.doi.org/10.1186/1472-6939-14-30]

[7]   Sanchini V BG, Disalvatore D, Monturano M, *et al.* A Trust-Based Pact in Research Biobanks. From Theory to Practice. Bioethics 2016; 30(4): 260-71.

[8]   Rasheed ZA, Kowalski J, Smith BD, Matsui W. Concise review: emerging concepts in clinical targeting of cancer stem cells. Stem Cells 2011; 29: 883-7.
[http://dx.doi.org/10.1002/stem.648] [PMID: 21509907]

CHAPTER 5

Rights and Obligations of Different Stakeholders Involved in Access and Use of Samples and Data in Biomedical Research[1]

Michiel Verlinden[1,*]**, Herman Nys**[2] **and Isabelle Huys**[3]

[1] *Clinical Pharmacology and Pharmacotherapy, KU Leuven, Belgium*

[2] *Interfaculty Centre for Biomedical Ethics and Law, KU Leuven, Belgium*

[3] *Centre for Intellectual Property Rights, KU Leuven, Belgium*

Abstract: Millions of human biological samples and associated data are collected each year for a variety of purposes. These purposes may include basic research, clinical trials and epidemiological studies. The legal framework that determines access to biobanks remains presently unclear. The absence of a defined set of applicable rules on international, European and national level creates legal uncertainty for biobanks and applicants. This chapter reports on four studies concerning the legal structure applicable to "Access to Biobanks". The first study consisted of a comparative analysis of access arrangements of organizations, biobank networks and biorepositories. The second study included interviews to gather qualitative data on the different perspectives held by stakeholders and experts in relation to the rights and obligations of custodians and applicants with respect to access to HBM and data stored in biobanks. The third study focused on the analysis of the legal framework applicable to access to biobanks. The final study (four) analysed the intellectual property rights (IPRs) in biobanking and the return and sharing of research results. These studies allowed us to formulate recommendations on the improvement of the legal framework applicable to public and private biobanks.

Keywords: Access, Biobank, Custodianship, Intellectual property, Legal framework.

INTRODUCTION

The European Strategy Forum on Research Infrastructures (ESFRI) identified biobanks as one of the main priority research infrastructures for the European Research Area (ERA) for the next 10 to 20 years [1, 2]. The 'Biobanking and

---

[*] **Corresponding author M. Verlinden:** Clinical Pharmacology and Pharmacotherapy, KU Leuven, Belgium; E-mail: michiel.verlinden@pharm.kuleuven.be

Elena Salvaterra and Julie Corfield (Eds.)
All rights reserved-© 2017 Bentham Science Publishers

Biomolecular resources Research Infrastructure' (BBMRI) was one of the first projects established under the European Research Infrastructure Preparatory Phase of ESFRI [3, 4]. The European Commission recognized the sound governance of biobanks as one of the most important challenges for the European innovation system [5].

For more than 100 years, millions of samples of human biological material (HBM) and associated data were collected in biobanks for a variety of purposes. These purposes included, for instance, basic research studies, clinical trials and epidemiological studies [6 - 8].

The exact definition of 'biobank' differs across countries. In Belgium for instance, article 2, 27° of the Belgian Act on HBM of 19 December 2008 defines a biobank as: "a structure that obtains, processes, stores and provides human bodily material and possible also associated data and *this (only) for scientific research purposes,* excluding research that implies medical applications to humans." (underlining by the authors). The rise of new scientific disciplines, such as genomics, proteomics and bioinformatics and new sequencing technologies in association with the initiative of precision medicine (PM) [9] considerably increased the demand for the systematic collection of large amounts of high quality human biological material (HBM) and data [3, 4]. The use and access to HBM and data stored in public biobanks has therefore become a crucial component in many biomedical research projects [10, 12].

Collections of HBM and data vary in scope, form and scale, according to the type of HBM and data that are retrieved and the different purposes for which they are used [13]. The scale ranges from small collections in hospital or university departments to the storage of large amounts of HBM in specifically designed and well-equipped facilities publicly or privately funded [8, 14].

Access to large amounts of HBM and data is crucial for many biomedical research projects. That is why several initiatives have been taken to develop biobank networks to share and combine different collections of HBM and data. The concept of a 'biobank network' can be defined as *'a group of institutions who freely assume the commitment to collaborate in the domain of biobanking and who (often) share the same procedures and quality policies, and who are (or might be) helped by a central hub for coordination in terms of service' [15].*

Different aspects determine the value of a biobank or biobank network. The quality of the samples and associated data and the ability to link the samples with donor information are two of these factors [16].

In the realm of translational research, biobanks and biobank networks will take a central place in the R&D process of medicines. Biobanks can provide a crucial platform for international and interdisciplinary cooperation and act "as key drivers for next generation biomarker (diagnostics) research and drug discovery" [17]. Good functioning models for access to HBM and data are crucial.

The legal framework that determines access to biobanks or biobank networks often remains unclear. The absence of a defined set of applicable rules creates legal uncertainty for biobanks and applicants. Our study investigated the hopes and concerns of the different stakeholders focusing on custodians of public biobanks and public and private applicants in biobanking. It mapped and characterized the present heterogeneous legal framework applicable to biobanks and formulated recommendations for the development of transparent, feasible and encouraging legal rules suitable for access to biobanks and biobank networks.The authors define custodianship as the "caretaking responsibility for HBM and data that starts at the planning of a biobank initiative, prior to the collection, and continues through research use to final dissemination of research results" (a slight adapted version of the definition used by R. Yassin *et al.* and the National Cancer Institute [34]).

Access Conditions to Biobanks and Biobank Networks

Theoretical and empirical research methods were designed and used to perform the studies [18 - 20] reported in this chapter, including literature reviews, interviews and in-depth document analyses.

A comparative document analysis of access arrangements of organizations, biobank networks and public as well private biobanks [19] is described here. This analysis provides qualitative data on the extent to which access arrangements contain information on selected access conditions. It furthermore considered to which extent access arrangements implement those access conditions in a harmonized way.

Furthemore, a comparative study of the legal framework that is applicable to access to biobanks [18] is described. This comparative study started with a general overview of the national legislation applicable to biobanks in Belgium and Denmark and legal norms at the international level and at the level of the Council of Europe. It also analyzed the rights and obligations of custodians of biobanks, applicants and - to a lesser extent– donors in these different legal instruments.

The last study reported in this chapter [20] entails a legal analysis of intellectual property rights (IPRs) in biobanking and to a lesser extent the return and sharing of research results. This study provides an overview of the most relevant IPRs in biobanking and discusses the risks and opportunities associated with the identified

IPRs for an effective protection and use of biobanks in translational research and innovation. It furthermore touches upon the question whether biobanks should require the return and sharing of research results.

Custodianship on HBM and Data Stored in Biobanks

Interviews were used to gain a more in-depth understanding on how access arrangements [19] are applied in the daily practice of biobank initiatives. The first part of the interview study focused on the *evaluation of access requests by access committees*. REC (Research Ethics Committee), access committees and possibly also funding bodies evaluate research projects from public and private applicants that request access to collections of HBM and data.

The interviews raised the importance of clarifying the interaction between those different entities [21]. There was no consensus among the interviewees on whether and to which extent access committees of biobanks should evaluate the quality, the scientific and medical usefulness and the ethical value of research projects. The existing legislation does not contain any guidance in this respect [18]. The interviewees did agree that access committees should only evaluate access requests on the condition that they dispose of sufficient expertise, experience and independence [6, 21 - 23]. Two interviewees with a legal background posed the question whether some or all of the evaluation criteria should be determined by binding legislation. They furthermore highlighted that the criteria should be equitable and proportionate. The legal study [18] revealed that the Best Practice 7.4 of the OECD Guidelines for Human Biobanks and Genetic Research Databases stipulates in this respect that custodians "need ensure that any stratified access or fees policies are fair, transparent and do no inhibit research" [24]. There was a consensus among the interviewees that equal access conditions should apply to internal and external academic applicants and non-academic private applicants.

Historically many clinicians and researchers created their own collections of HBM and data. The analysis in Verlinden *et al*, 2014 [19] revealed a trend to assign in access arrangements custodianship to biobanks or biobank networks and no longer to individual collectors or principal investigators. This can be explained by the fact that biomedical research requires access to large amounts of HBM and data of high quality [22, 25 - 27].

Finally, the comparative document analysis confirmed that the majority of the biobank initiatives establishes an access committee to evaluate requests for access to HBM and data [19].

The informants seem to agree that the custodian of the biobank has the right to take the final decision on *whether leftover HBM should be returned or destroyed*. However, the interviews demonstrated the difficulty to determine generally applicable criteria on whether the biobank should request the return or destruction of leftover HBM. The comparative document analysis and other previous studies confirmed that biobanks apply different policies on leftover HBM [12, 18]. Following the interviews, there is however no doubt that applicants need to obtain an approval of the (access committee of a) biobank – and a research ethics committee – to use leftover HBM in another project.

With respect to the access fees charged by biobanks, interviewees considered those fees as often insufficient to compensate all costs in relation to the collection, storage and distribution of HBM and data for research purposes. New mechanisms need to be developed to feed some of the benefits of biomedical research back into the biobank infrastructure and the health care system [22, 29].

The interviewees were rather sceptical about the idea that providers of HBM and associated data should be able to participate in downstream IPRs or royalties on such IPRs. Following the study on IPRs and biobanking [20] biobanks should only be involved in downstream IPRs if they made a (intellectual or scientific/technical) contribution to the results of a research project.

The interviewees suggest that public biobanks might charge a higher access fee to industrial applicants – compared to academic applicants – for access to a publicly funded collection of HBM and data [11, 30]. This could be justified by the fact that those collections have been created with public funding. The comparative document analysis [19] had already shown that several biobank initiatives apply different access fees depending on the type of applicant. However, the best practice guideline 7.4 of the OECD Guidelines stipulates that the custodian of a biobank has to ensure that any stratified access conditions and fees are fair, transparent and do not inhibit research [24].

There was consensus among the interviewees that an applicant could be required to share his research results with the biobank and/or other researchers. This is no surprise, since the majority of the access arrangements provided that a biobank could require the return and/or the sharing of research results [19]. One should however protect the legitimate interests of the researcher that generated the research results.

The OECD Guidelines for Human Biobanks and Genetic Research Databases suggest in this respect that a biobank should develop a policy on whether and how the results of research and analyses carried out using HBM and data stored in biobanks should be returned to the biobank.

Today, numerous collections of HBM and data are established at the initiative of the principal investigators of specific research projects. Furthermore biobanks still rely on individual clinicians or researchers for the collection of specific HBM and data. Biobank initiatives could recognize such contribution by granting a temporary priority right to conduct research with the collected HBM and data and to allow publication of the results [11, 23].

Legal Framework Governing Access and Use of HBM and Data for Research Purposes

The future Belgian legislation and the Danish legislation applicable to biobanks mainly focuses on the rights and obligations of the donor and the custodian [18]. The legal framework contains, for instance, quite detailed rules on the obligation to respect the informed consent of the donor and the protection of the personal data of the donor. The study of legal documents also revealed a considerable list of rights and obligations held by the custodian of a biobank. Finally several legal documents stipulate that a REC or another competent authority should review the aims and activities of a biobank. Fewer provisions relate to the rights and obligations of the applicants.

The Belgian and Danish legislation applicable to biobanks contain specific rules on the review of access requests by ethics committees. It does not provide anything in relation to the mandate of an access committee. Some international normative instruments do provide additional guidance on the role of an access committee and the development of access policies, procedures and mechanisms [18]. The OECD Guidelines for Human Biobanks and Genetic Research Databases [24] formulate a general principle on the development of biobanks policies. They express the principle that public biobanks should develop policies on the commercialization of HBM and data, IPRs, the sharing in scientific advancements and its benefits and the sharing of research results. They do not contain concrete guidance on how to develop such policies. The interviews reported in the previous paragraph revealed that no consensus exists among biobank initiatives on how to develop a policy on IPRs and benefit sharing.

IPRS In Biobanking: Challenges and Opportunities for Translational Research

Both the comparative analysis of access arrangements [19] and the interviews confirm that the majority of the public biobank initiatives did not develop any policy in relation to IPRs. This might be explained by the fact that the existence and especially the exercise of IPRs in relation to HBM and data have been found controversial in the past. The exclusive nature of IPRs could also be considered incompatible with the need to facilitate access to public biobanks [31]. An IPR policy may just as well be used as a tool to enhance the acknowledgement and protection of the interests of the biobank and to stimulate the development of biobanks as essential research tools or infrastructures [32]. One should however avoid ending up in a situation in which IPRs would constitute an obstacle to the use of HBM and data in research projects.

Our study [20] highlights the main challenges and suggests possible strategies and options with regard to this topic. It tackles the question of how to address and manage IPRs directed to HBM, the associated data stored in the biobank and the results of research using the HBM and associated data. We looked amongst others into the question whether biobanks should be involved in upstream and downstream IPRs. Finally the study highlights how biobanks could be involved in the development of policies on the sharing of research results. We also suggest developing policies to ensure an increased recognition of the contributions of biobanks and collectors to research projects.

Harmonization Across Biobank Initiatives

The comparative analysis of access arrangements revealed a lack of harmonization on how access conditions are defined and implemented [19] both in public and private biobanks. This lack of harmonization can be explained by the fact that the concepts of 'biobanks' and 'biobank networks' represent a heterogeneous group of infrastructures that collect various types of HBM and data. Some discrepancies could also be explained by the various approaches on ethical and legal issues in biobanking in the different countries [22]. This heterogeneity in access conditions makes it questionably whether one should provide 'one size fits all' conditions on access to (public) biobanks [15]. Attempts to harmonise access conditions could focus on particular types of biobanks, such as tumour or stem cell banks or population-based biobanks. In another approach they could focus on rather technical issues, such as quality standards or minimum data sets.

Harmonization could also focus on specific access conditions, such as IPRs, the sharing of research results [33] and non-financial benefit sharing. The interviews and the legal study [18] confirmed that such specific conditions are not yet harmonized. Finally, attention could be given to some other biobank initiatives (such as OECD and P^{3}G), which did not attempt to harmonize access rules, but rather to develop best practices or guidelines. Such best practices [24, 34 - 37] or guidelines do not suggest a uniform set of rules. They aim to provide a general (legal) framework that can be used as inspiration for the creation of access rules within other biobank initiatives. In this way they may indirectly stimulate harmonisation.

Does the Existing Legal Framework Regulate the Key Access Conditions?

The aforementioned access policy document analysis revealed that several "key access conditions" are regulated by the majority of the studied access arrangements, such as (1) the level of custodianship; (2) the establishment of access committees; and (3) the mandate of such access committees.

We concluded from the interviews that a number of "key access conditions" would preferably be regulated *via* access arrangements, such as (1) the access conditions and fees that apply to industrial and external applicants; (2) priority setting; (3) priority access for collectors of HBM and data; and (4) the return and destruction of leftover HBM.

The study on the legal framework revealed that other "key access conditions" are mainly regulated *via* legislation or soft law, in particular: (1) the review of the aims, activities and policies of biobanks by RECs; (2) the rights and obligations of custodians; (3) the review of access requests by REC; (4) the principle that one should not generate profit on HBM (as such); (5) data protection; (6) consent.

A limited number of 'key access conditions" seem to be insufficiently regulated *via* the existing legal framework, in particular: (1) the sharing or returning of research results; (2) benefit sharing; and (3) intellectual property.

Many different players and instruments determine the legal conditions for access to biobanks. National legislation, international normative instruments and access arrangements each play a distinct role in the regulation of access to biobanks. Access arrangements do not need to contain specific rules on legal issues that are already sufficiently regulated by national legislation or international normative instruments (or soft law). The protection of personal data is a good example of an issue that access arrangements do not have to deal with in detail given the well-developed international, European and national legislation in this regard. Another issue that is regulated in detail by legislation and soft law is the requirement to obtain the informed consent of the donor for the removal, the storage and/or the use of HBM and data for research purposes. On the other hand, the existing legislation and soft law does not provide any guidance on how to calculate financial and material compensations for operations conducted with HBM and data. Here, guidance in access arrangements could provide an additional tool to avoid the commercialization of HBM.

Taking into account the heterogeneous nature of biobanks, legislation should not over-regulate access to biobanks. That is why we doubt, for instance, whether national legislation or international normative documents should regulate the requirement to return or destroy leftover HBM. One could also doubt whether the evaluation of access requests by access committees should be regulated in detail by national legislation or international normative instruments. Some aspects of access to biobanks could be regulated *via* codes of conduct, guidelines and best practices. Those instruments could, for instance, be used to develop policies on (1) priority access of collectors of HBM and data; (2) the sharing or returning of research results; (3) benefit sharing; and (4) intellectual property. The advantage of such instruments is that they are created after consultation with the different stakeholders involved in biobanking. Such instruments may also be more easily adaptable in order to take new technological or biomedical evolutions into account. Although they are not enforceable as national legislation, they do have an important influence. An example of this is the Code of Conduct developed in the Netherlands by FEDERA – the Dutch Federation of Medical Scientific Societies – and COREON – the Commission on Regulation in Research –. It was produced in close collaboration with the Dutch Patient Consumer Federation, the Federation of Parent and Patient Organisations and BBMRI-NL. This Code of Conduct contains relatively detailed rules and principles on how to deal in a responsible manner with HBM (and data) in the context of health research [42]. The Code of Conduct created a certain extent of harmonization, since many biobanks, biobank networks and organizations in the Netherlands committed to respect this common set of rules and principles. Other important access arrangements have been developed by the National Cancer Institute in the US [34], ISBER [43], the OECD [24, 35] and P³G [36, 37].

Biobanks Should Develop Clear Policies on the Evaluation of Access Requests

A considerable number of access arrangements [19] did not contain transparent information on how public biobank initiatives implement several of the studied access conditions. The lack of clear information on access conditions could hinder access to biobanks and biobank networks [9, 11, 26, 25, 36, 38 - 41].

Public biobanks should provide publicly available information about their access arrangements and procedures [24, 44]. Access arrangements should clarify the mandate of access committees. They should in particular specify which criteria and procedures will be applied in the evaluation of access requests [6, 11, 21, 24]. The procedure for the evaluation of access requests should protect the interests of the donor and the biobank. It should, for instance, avoid that HBM and data is wasted on research projects of insufficient quality. It should not, however, become unnecessarily burdensome. For instance, an access committee should not evaluate the same criteria as a REC and/or a data protection authority. Access arrangements could clarify how access committees will supplement the mandatory evaluations by REC or other competent authorities [5].

When an access committee evaluates access requests and the scientific merits of applicants, it needs to make sure that it possesses of the necessary competence to make such evaluations. In some cases, it may be advisable to consult external reviewers in the evaluation of certain access requests.

Access arrangements should contain clear instructions on which information an applicant needs to provide in his research protocol [24]. One could refer in this respect to the Good Clinical Practices that are applied in clinical trials. They could constitute a source of inspiration.

Access arrangements should stipulate to which extent certain types of research will be given priority [24]. One could for instance imagine that diseases-oriented biobanks would prioritize research that corresponds with their own core field of interest.

Access arrangements should clearly specify the rights and obligations of the custodian, the applicant and the donor in relation to the collection and disposition of HBM and data.

Finally, one should avoid 'restrictive' access arrangements that would limit access to collections of HBM and data and as consequence would unnecessarily hamper the development of biomedical research.

Define the Conditions for Access by Industrial Companies

The majority of the biobank initiatives agree that industrial companies – such as pharmaceutical and biotechnological companies – can access and use HBM and data from publicly funded biobanks. Industrial companies play an important role in the transformation of research into a drug candidate and eventually into a medical product. However, access by industrial companies should not have a negative impact on the donors' trust and willingness to provide HBM and data to biobanks [45]. That is why biobank initiatives should clearly communicate about their relationships with industrial companies. It would be desirable to clearly define the conditions under which industrial companies can access publicly funded collections of HBM and data. Those conditions could be developed in consultation with the different stakeholders, such as the funders of the biobanks, the donors and the applicants.

Recognize the Contribution of Individual Collectors

The comparative analysis of access arrangements and the interviews confirmed that custodianship over HBM and data has shifted over time from individual collectors to biobanks. However, individual collectors still make important contributions to the collections of HBM and associated data. Individual collectors could also provide important know how on the HBM and associated data. Proper incentives should be given to the individual collectors and their contributions [5]. It could be envisioned to grant certain collectors a temporary priority right to conduct research with the collected HBM and data and to publish the results [11, 23]. It is considered good practice to inform the collectors of HBM and data, when such HBM and data is used in research projects. One should however investigate the practical implications of such practice. It may be a good idea to also consult individual collectors in the decision to make HBM and data available for a specific research project. This does not imply a veto right for the individual collector. The final decision to distribute HBM and associated data remains with the custodian of the biobank.

Develop Policy on Sharing of Research Results

Previous studies confirmed that an increasing number of public biobanks [28] and funding bodies [46] require researchers to make their research results publicly available. Such requirement is motivated by the desire to maximize the use of results of publicly funded research [47, 48]. Some authors also invoke the principle of reciprocity. Researchers could be expected to share their results with stakeholders that contributed to the collection of HBM and data, such as biobanks and donors [23, 49]. However, the sharing of research results will only be useful and acceptable for researchers if the following three conditions are fulfilled. First, the proper infrastructure needs to be available to store and allow other researchers access to the research results [47]. Second, the conditions under which other researchers can access the results should be clearly defined. Finally, it should be taken into account that researchers could have a legitimate interest to request that some research results remain confidential. This is necessary to allow the researchers to publish their results and possibly obtain IPRs on clinical applications based on those results [21, 23, 47, 49, 50].

Develop Policy on Intellectual Property Rights

IPR policies could constitute an important tool to protect the considerable investments made in the creation of collections of HBM and data. Such policies will only be successful if the interest and concerns of the different stakeholders are respected [51]. Transparency towards the donors is important. The donors should be aware of the possibility of obtaining and exercising IPRs in relation to the collection of HBM and data. The policy should contain clear information on which IPRs the biobank (or the collecting researchers) might claim in relation to the collection of HBM and data. It should also be clear which IPRs the potential users can hold in relation to research results obtained from using HBM and data.

Unless the biobank made an important (intellectual or scientific) contribution to the results of a research project, it could be useful for them to focus on the protection of their upstream IPRs and not on downstream IPRs. A proper policy on downstream IPRs should encourage applicants/researchers but also biobanks not to obtain excessive IPRs. The policy should however contain sufficient incentives to innovate. Applicants have a legitimate interest to obtain IPRs on downstream clinical applications or products [52]. Basic upstream data, research tools and enabling technologies should, however, remain available to the scientific community [32, 37, 53]. Finally, we suggest revising international guidelines on co-authorship to clarify which type of contributions could result in co-authorship. Such new guidelines could recognize more essential technical or scientific contributions to research projects [54]. Alternatively, biobank policies could clarify how contributions to research projects would be recognized and rewarded [11, 23, 50].

Involve Donors and Patients in the Biobank Policy

The future evolution of biobanks depends to a large extent on the willingness of donors to provide HBM and data for biomedical research. That is why (public) biobanks need to make sure that they maintain the trust of those donors. The interests and concerns of donors and patients should be taken into account in every aspect of a biobank policy [45]. Biobanks should maintain an open dialogue with the donors about their activities and policies. Finally it is important to create more public awareness of the important contributions of biobanks to biomedical research and innovation [5].

Future Perspectives

In this chapter it is questioned whether the existing legal framework corresponds to the needs of public biobanks and other stakeholders, in particular non academic private industries.

We quickly came to realize that the concepts of 'biobanks' and 'biobank networks' represent a heterogeneous group of infrastructures. It is therefore not so straightforward to formulate uniform rules on access to biobanks in general.

We also noticed that the discipline of biobanking is still relatively young [30] Many countries are developing new biobank infrastructures. This might explain why several access arrangements of biobank initiatives did not contain information on several key access conditions. Many biobanks initiatives will continue to develop their access arrangements. One can refer in this respect to recent initiatives of, for instance, P^{3}G [36, 37]. Some (public) biobank initiatives increasingly exchange experiences on practical matters related to biobanking but also on legal knowledge.

In November 2014 BBMRI-ERIC announced the creation of a European Centre for Ethical, Legal and Social Issues (ELSI) on biobanking. One can expect that this will generate new opportunities to develop codes of conduct, guidelines or best practices, and routines for access to biobanks. Those opportunities might even lead to an increased harmonisation of the European legal framework applicable to biobanks. In addition, BBMRI-ERIC has initiated a Stakeholder Forum to align interests of different stakeholders in the context of biobanking.

As previously seen [18], the legal framework on biobanks is still evolving. With respect to the Belgian situation, one can refer to the fact that the future provisions on biobanks in the Belgian Act on HBM still have not entered into force. The Belgian Minister of Health, furthermore, announced in her policy note that the provisions on biobanks will further be developed and improved in consultation with the stakeholders.

Taken into account the evolving nature of biobanks, we hope that this chapter can be inspiring to these recent legal developments and may contribute to the creation of a clear and smooth legal framework on access to public and private biobanks.

NOTES

[1] This chapter was drafted on the basis of studies conducted in the framework of a PhD project funded by the Agency for Innovation by Science and Technology in Flanders (Belgium) (IWT).

CONFLICT OF INTEREST

The authors confirm that they have no conflict of interest to declare for this publication.

ACKNOWLEDGEMENT

Declared none.

REFERENCES

[1]   Biological and Medical Sciences; Roadmap Working Group. Report 2008. Brussels 2008.

[2]   Report of the Expert Group on Research Infrastructures: A vision for strengthening world class research infrastructures on the ERA 2010.

[3]   Asslaber M, Zatloukal K. Biobanks: transnational, European and global networks. In: Zatloukal K, Ed. Brief Funct Genomic Proteomic. , Austria: Institute of Pathology, Medical University of Graz, A-8036 Graz 2007; 6: pp. [cited 2014 Mar 4];(3)193-201.

[4]   Yuille M, van Ommen G-J, Brechot C, *et al.* Biobanking for Europe. In: Yuille M, Ed. Brief

Bioinform. United Kingdom: The University of Manchester, School of Translational Medicine, CIGMR, Manchester M13 9PT 2008; 9: pp. (1)14-24.

[5]   Biobanks for Europe. A challenge for governance. Luxembourg 2012.

[6]   Vaught J, Lockhart NC. The evolution of biobanking best practices. Clin Chim Acta 2012; 413(19-20): 1569-75.
[http://dx.doi.org/10.1016/j.cca.2012.04.030]

[7]   Czerepak E a. Drug approvals and failures: implications for alliances. Nat Rev Drug Discov 2008; 7(3): 197-8.

[8]   Vaught JB, Henderson MK, Compton CC. Biospecimens and biorepositories: from afterthought to science. Cancer Epidemiol Biomarkers Prev 2012; 21(2): 253-5.
[http://dx.doi.org/10.1158/1055-9965.EPI-11-1179]

[9]   Precision Medicine

[10]   Meir K, Gaffney EF, Simeon-Dubach D, *et al.* The human face of biobank networks for translational research. Biopreserv Biobank 2011; 9(3): 279-85.
[http://dx.doi.org/10.1089/bio.2011.0018] [PMID: 24850340]

[11]   Fortin S, Pathmasiri S, Grintuch R, *et al.* Deschenes M. "Access arrangements" for biobanks: a fine line between facilitating and hindering collaboration. Public Health Genomics. P3G Consortium, Montreal, QC H3V 1A2, Canada 2011; 14: pp. (2)104-4.

[12]   Edwards T, Cadigan RJ, Evans JP, *et al.* Biobanks containing clinical specimens: defining characteristics, policies, and practices. Clin Biochem Elsevier BV 2014; 47(4-5): 245-51.
[http://dx.doi.org/10.1016/j.clinbiochem.2013.11.023]

[13]   Gottweis H, Zatloukal K. Biobank governance: trends and perspectives. Pathobiology 2007; 74(4): 206-11.
[http://dx.doi.org/10.1159/000104446]

[14]   Advice no 45 of 19 January 2009 concerning banks of human bodily material for research purposes 2009.

[15]   Morente MM, Cereceda L, Luna-Crespo F, Artiga MJ. Managing a biobank network. Biopreserv Biobank 2011; 9(2): 187-90.
[http://dx.doi.org/10.1089/bio.2011.0005] [PMID: 24846266]

[16]   Bell WC, Sexton KC, Grizzle WE. Organizational issues in providing high-quality human tissues and clinical information for the support of biomedical research. Methods Mol Biol 2010; 576: 1-30.

[17]   Hasan S. The Increasing Role of Biobanks in Personalized Medicine [Internet]

[18]   Verlinden M. Legal framework applicable to access to biobanks 2015.

[19]   Verlinden M, Nys H, Ectors N, *et al.* Access to biobanks: harmonization across biobank initiatives. Biopreserv Biobank 2014; 12(6): 415-22.
[http://dx.doi.org/10.1089/bio.2014.0034]

[20]   Verlinden M, Minssen T, Huys I. IPRs in biobanking : risks and opportunities for translational research. Intellect Prop Q 2015; 1(2): 106-29.

[21]   Shabani M, Knoppers BM, Borry P. From the principles of genomic data sharing to the practices of data access committees. EMBO Mol Med 2015; 7(5): 507-9.
[http://dx.doi.org/10.15252/emmm.201405002] [PMID: 25759363]

[22]   Cambon-Thomsen A, Rial-Sebbag E, Knoppers BM. Trends in ethical and legal frameworks for the use of human biobanks. Eur Respir J 2007; 30(2): 373-82.
[http://dx.doi.org/10.1183/09031936.00165006]

[23]   Mascalzoni D, Dove ES, Rubinstein Y, *et al.* International Charter of principles for sharing bio-specimens and data. Eur J Hum Genet 1] Center for Research Ethics and Bioethics Uppsala

University, Uppsala, Sweden [2] Center for Biomedicine, EURAC Research, Bolzano, Italy Centre of Genomics and Policy, Mc Gill University, Montreal, Quebec, Canada Office for Rare Diseases Research, Natio 2014. (1476-5438 (Electronic))

[24]   OECD Guidelines on Human Biobanks and Genetic Research Databases. Eur J Health Law 2009 p; 191-204.

[25]   O'Brien SJ. Stewardship of human biospecimens, DNA, genotype, and clinical data in the GWAS era. Annu Rev Genomics Hum Genet 2009; 10(May): 193-209.

[26]   Lemrow SM, Colditz GA, Vaught JB, *et al.* Key elements of access policies for biorepositories associated with population science research. Cancer Epidemiol Biomarkers Prev 2007; 16(8): 1533-5. [http://dx.doi.org/10.1158/1055-9965.EPI-07-0101]

[27]   Bauer K, Taub S, Parsi K. Ethical issues in tissue banking for research: a brief review of existing organizational policies. Theor Med Bioeth 2004; 25(2): 113-42. [http://dx.doi.org/10.1023/B:META.0000033772.84738.ad]

[28]   Henderson GE, Edwards TP, Cadigan RJ, *et al.* Stewardship practices of U.S. biobanks. Sci Transl Med 2013; 5(215): 1-6. [http://dx.doi.org/10.1126/scitranslmed.3007362] [PMID: 24337477]

[29]   Bovenberg J. Whose tissue is it anyway? Nat Biotechnol 2005; 23(8): 929-33. [http://dx.doi.org/10.1038/nbt0805-929] [PMID: 16082356]

[30]   Riegman PHJ, Morente MM, Betsou F, *et al.* Biobanking for better healthcare. Mol Oncol Riegman, PHJ, Department of Pathology, Josephine Nefkens Institute, Erasmus Medical Center, 3015 GE Rotterdam, Netherlands 2008; 2(3): 213-2. [http://dx.doi.org/10.1016/j.molonc.2008.07.004]

[31]   Dove ES, Joly Y. The contested futures of biobanks and intellectual property. Teoría y derecho 2012; 11: 132-47.

[32]   Pénin J, Wack J-P. Research tool patents and free-libre biotechnology: A suggested unified framework. Res Policy 2008; 37(10): 1909-21. [http://dx.doi.org/10.1016/j.respol.2008.07.012]

[33]   International Code of Conduct for Genomic and Health-Related Data Sharing 2014.

[34]   NCI Best Practices for Biospecimen Resources [Internet] 2011. Available from: http://biospecimens.cancer.gov/bestpractices/2011-NCIBestPractices.pdf

[35]   OECD Best Practices Guidelines for Biological Resource Centres 2007.

[36]   Knoppers BM, Chisholm RL, Kaye J, *et al.* A P3G generic access agreement for population genomic studies. Nat Biotechnol Nature Publishing Group 2013; 31(5): 384-5.

[37]   Knoppers BM, Chisholm RL, Kaye J, *et al.* P3G Model Framework for Biobank Governance. Nat Biotechnol Montreal 2013; 31(5): 384-5.

[38]   Access to collections of data and materials for health research: A report to the Medical Research Council and the Wellcome Trust [Internet]. Medical Research Council and the Wellcome Trust 2006. Available from:http://www.wellcome.ac.uk/About-us/Publications/Reports/Biomedical-ethics/WTX0 30843. htm120

[39]   Vaught J, Kelly A, Hewitt R. A review of international biobanks and networks: Success factors and key benchmarks. Biopreserv Biobank. In: Vaught J, Ed. Office of Biorepositories and Biospecimen Research (OBBR), National Cancer Institute, National Institutes of Health, Bethesda, MD 20892, United States. 2009; 7: pp. (3)143-50.

[40]   Joly Y, Zeps N, Knoppers BM. Genomic databases access agreements: legal validity and possible sanctions. Hum Genet 2011; 25;130(3): 441-9. [http://dx.doi.org/10.1007/s00439-011-1044-3]

[41] Colledge F, Elger B, Howard HC. A Review of the Barriers to Sharing in Biobanking. Biopreserv Biobank , 2013 [cited 2014 Jan 17];11(6): 339-46. [http://dx.doi.org/10.1089/bio.2013.0039]

[42] Human tissue and medical research. Code of conduct for responsible use. 2011.

[43] Campbell LD, Betsou F, Garcia DL, *et al.* Development of the ISBER best practices for repositories: collection, storage, retrieval and distribution of biological materials for research. Biopreserv Biobank 2012; 10(2): 232-3.

[44] Working document on research on biological materials of human origin. Strasbourg: Committee on Bioethics 2014 p. 10.

[45] Minssen T, Schovsbo J. Legal aspects of biobanking as key issues for personalized medicine and translational exploitation. Per Med 2014; 11(5): 497-508. [http://dx.doi.org/10.2217/pme.14.29]

[46] Kosseim P, Dove ES, Baggaley C, *et al.* Building a data sharing model for global genomic research. Genome Biol 2014; 15(8): 430. [http://dx.doi.org/10.1186/s13059-014-0430-2]

[47] Knoppers BM, Harris JR, Tassé AM, *et al.* Towards a data sharing code of conduct for international genomic research. Genome Med 2011; 3(7): 46. [http://dx.doi.org/10.1186/gm262] [PMID: 21787442]

[48] Ness RB. Biospecimen "ownership": point. Cancer Epidemiol Biomarkers Prev 2007; 16(2): 188-9. [http://dx.doi.org/10.1158/1055-9965.EPI-06-1011]

[49] Boggio A. Transfer of samples and sharing of results: requirements imposed on researchers. In: Elger BS, Biller-Andorno N, Mauron A, Eds. Ethical and regulatory aspects of human genetic databases. Ashgate 2008; pp. 1-11.

[50] Framework for Responsible Sharing of Genomic and Health-Related Data [Internet]. Global Alliance for Genomics and Health 2013. Available from: http://genomicsandhealth.org/framework

[51] Heaney C, Carbone J, Gold R, *et al.* The perils of taking property too far. Stanf J Law Sci Policy 2009; 1: 46-64.

[52] Pathmasiri S, Deschênes M, Joly Y, *et al.* Intellectual property rights in publicly funded biobanks: much ado about nothing? Nat Biotechnol. Nature Publishing Group 2011; 29(4): 319-23. [http://dx.doi.org/10.1038/nbt.1834]

[53] Simon BM, Law S, Barton J, *et al.* How to get a fair share: IP policies for publicly supported biobanks. Stanf J Law Sci Policy 2008; 452(2003): 65-79.

[54] Colledge FM, Elger BS, Shaw DM, *et al.* "Conferring authorship": biobank stakeholders' experiences with publication credit in collaborative research. PLoS One 2013 Jan 2013; 8(9): e76686.

CHAPTER 6

HUB Organization to Enhance Access to Biological Resources: a French Example

Jeanne-Hélène di Donato[1,*] and **Pascal Auré**[2]

[1] *3C-R, Biobank Consulting Company, 1 Impasse des Pinsons 31780 Castelginest, France*

[2] *BioTechBANK, 18 rue Proust, 49100 Angers, France*

Abstract: The main purpose of biobanks is to provide private and public organisations with biological resources to be used for research projects but unfortunately this process is often not straightforward. Most biobanks supply biological resources to research teams within their own organizations and have difficulty in supplying samples to external teams. The most difficult step is to obtain a specific collaboration agreement between the two parties. This step takes a long time and often interferes with research planning. Moreover, most of French biobanks are administered and financed by hospitals or public research institutes, which established the biobanks for the purpose of supporting their own researchers. The supply of biological resources in the absence of scientific collaboration was not a part of the original plan. Yet today these biobanks need to supply research teams in private/commercial organisations, to promote the use of their samples, to develop translational research and to obtain a return on investment. The rights and needs of researchers must be take into account but priority must be given to the valorization of the biobank. To encourage optimal use of samples and avoid the costly conservation of unused collections, we propose a "HUB" organization to enhance access to biological resources in France. The development of this organization and drafting of legal agreements must take into account the following considerations: a) the researchers' current needs must be fully understood: this depends on excellent communications between the HUB and legal representatives of the research teams, and b) the availability of collections through a biobank network must be fully understood: this depends on excellent communications between the HUB and legal representatives of the biobanks.

Keywords: Biobanks, Biobank sustainability, Biological resource centres, Collection, Contract, MTA, Public-private collaboration, Supply.

INTRODUCTION

Research in academia and industry often requires large sets of biological samples to develop new programs or to validate a scientific concept. The process of

* Corresponding author Jeanne-Hélène di Donato: 3C-R, 1 Impasse des Pinsons, 31780 Castelginest, France; Tel: 09 75 20 9321 E-mail: jhdd@3cr-ressourcesbiologiques.com

Elena Salvaterra and Julie Corfield (Eds.)
All rights reserved-© 2017 Bentham Science Publishers

obtaining sufficient samples that meet quality criteria defined by international standards is often time-consuming for researchers and reduces their competitiveness. In response to their needs biobanks have been developed over the past 20 years to manage sample collections under standard operating procedures and to ensure that the quality and ethical requirements of international recommendations [1, 2] and national regulations are met. So, gradually, biobanks have become an important provider of biological resources for researchers [3, 4].

However, in general biobanks have focused more on ensuring sample quality by efficient collection and storage of materials, and less on the efficient distribution of samples to researchers. This is a consequence of the fact that most biobanks distribute samples to researchers who initially collected samples (clinicians) or at least to researchers who are linked to the biobank in some way (*i.e*, through a scientific relationship) as demonstrated by findings of the European report [5]. Even in the case of an open sharing policy, they usually give samples to academic teams without charging a fee for the service. Similarly, a study of US biobanks demonstrated that only 2% of them charge a fee for samples [6] and a Canadian study found that cost recovery ranged between 5%-25% of the actual cost [7]. This situation is due to the fact that most biobanks are financed by public funding or per-project funding [8].

Despite these models, the economic situation is more stringent globally and the cost of biobanking activities continues to grow. Academic biobanks need to be as competitive as commercial biobanks which usually develop business to meet the demands of pharmaceutical companies [9].

Even if some reports estimate that biorepositories can save millions in research funding [10], it is clear that biobanks today will need to find adequate and reliable sources of funding to be sustainable in the long-term [1, 11]. It is possible to have an optimistic view of biobanking development. Many repositories have very under-used collections, so by improving access to these collections we may be able to meet some of the growing demand for human biospecimens.

A return-on–investment policy is necessary to maintain the high quality of collections and ensure biobanks sustainability through a model which takes into account the relationship of altruism and solidarity between donors and biobanks [12]. There are more and more publications that present such models as business plans [13 - 16] and demonstrate that creating viable funding models is a pre-requisite for the sustainability of biobanks.

These developments encourage academic biobanks to face difficulties they must overcome to become sustainable. To this end, biobanks are involved in the development of tools such as catalogues [17], harmonised operating procedures

[18], and processes for request management to strengthen communication and promote demand. In the same way tables of costs have been established and published [19, 20] in order to provide biobanks with standard prices for services. Even though it is unethical to sell human samples, all the processes around collection, storage and supply of human samples can be costed. For example, the Canadian Tissue Repository network developed a tool to calculate the appropriate user fees [21]. In France, the billing policy for biobank services has been published in "Journal Officiel de la République Française" in a specific chapter on clinical activities.

Networks of biobanks can also contribute to sustainability as for example where a number of biobanks work together to add value to a collection [22]. Another type of biobank network, based on a Hub model might be particularly useful for enhancing sample exchange: according to this model a third party would act as a Hub, linking sample suppliers and sample requesters in a win-win collaboration.

The HUB MODEL

Initially developed by airline companies to improve traffic at the airport, the Hub concept is based on a central interface facilitating trade. In the case of research, some Hub organizations have been described which facilitate harmonization of sample management [23] and synergy between different partners [24]. The Hub solution has been explored in order to deal with the requests for samples and the wish to supply samples with the aim of quick movement of inputs (the requests for samples) and outputs (the supply of samples).

HUB-BTB-3CR is a Hub organisation developed by BioTech BANK and 3C-R. In this organisation, sample requests are managed centrally by a central node (the HUB) so that researchers working in the public or private domains can have direct access to all biobanks that belong to the HUB-BTB-3CR (Fig. 1).

HUB provides linkage between the researchers' needs (most of them are from pharmaceutical or biotechnology companies)and a network of biobanks which can provide them the samples. Through the HUB all the sample requests are shared with all the biobanks in order to provide the opportunity to match the needs of the two parties quickly. This model is particularly effective and useful in the case of requests for rare disease samples.

For the HUB-BTB-3C-Rorganisationto be successful, there are the following requirements:

- there must be a large number of biobanks able to respond quickly to requests,
- the researcher's needs must be well defined and well understood,

− there must be an effective agreement between the HUB and the stakeholders (legal entities of both the sample suppliers and the sample requesters),
− there must be an operating procedure to manage each request in total transparency.

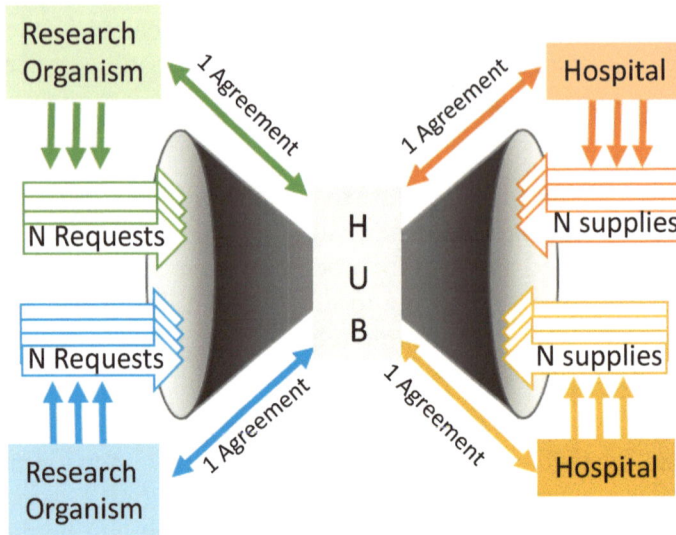

Fig. (1). Hub model to be efficient supplying biospecimens.

Relationship between Biobanks and the HUB

To be efficient, a Hub organization requires the involvement of numerous biobanks and the knowledge of their sample collections. There are already some well-known initiatives involving common catalogues to give information about the samples available at regional [25] or international [26, 27] levels, but most of these initiatives are specialized or non-exhaustive.

Besides the number of biobanks, another important success factor is the need for good communication with the biobanks to discuss precise needs and expectations of the researchers requesting the samples.

In the case of HUB-BTB-3CR, the biobanks rely on Club 3C-R [28], a private network of 89 French biobanks in the area of human health managed by one person who has a privileged relationship with each biobank. The database of this network identifies the main samples in terms of nature (tissue, DNA, cells…), preparation and preservation (fixed, cryopreserved, slides, buffy coat…) and diseases. The knowledge and experience that exists within this established network leads to increased efficiency, because requests are only sent to biobanks that are likely to respond. Preliminary biobank selection by the HUB avoids inappropriate and useless e-mails, which is greatly appreciated by the biobanks.

Relationship between Research Teams and the HUB

The development of personalised medicine depends on modern research in the area of human health [29, 30]. To develop knowledge of diagnostic biomarkers and appropriate treatments, research teams need access to well characterized collections. For this reason, biobanks are increasingly becoming translational research partners [31, 32]. To be efficient, it is essential to have rapid access to suitable samples. Initially, the HUB-BTB-3CR provides research teams with preliminary information about availability of samples in France. Then, if it seems likely that an identified biobank can meet a request, detailed discussions are initiated that involve the research team, the biobank and the HUB.

Simplification of the Agreement for Sharing Biospecimens

Sample supply must follow an agreement defining the rights and duties of each party. These agreements are written to protect the rights of each party, but they often create an administrative burden. The most difficult aspects include intellectual property issues, deciding cost-recovery fees for biobanks, general information about sample use, return of research results and acknowledgement of biobanks in publications [33]. But people representing the legal entities involved in developing these agreements are generally not as concerned as researchers by the deadlines and the need to generate these official documents quickly [34]. In context of competition, one of the challenges is the quick execution of a program. To overcome this difficulty, HUB-BTB-3CR proposes the development of a framework agreement between itself and legal entities of the biobanks and the research teams. This global agreement defines the general rules of collaboration under which biobanks can supply biological resources and there search teams can obtain them. Under this agreement, the legal entity delegates responsibility for each request to the Biobank Manager on one side and the Principal Researcher on the other.

Once the general contract has been signed, this system allows the people directly concerned to manage scientific and technical points both quickly and efficiently.

The traceability of requests and sample supply is then ensured by a signed quotation sent from the HUB representative to the researcher and biobank involved in each request.

Process of Request Management and Sample Supply

The request process (Fig. **2**) may be initiated once the framework agreement has been signed. Through the HUB-BTB-3C Rorganization each sample request is addressed to target biobanks which potentially have the samples. A strength of HUB-BTB-3CR is being able to contact biobanks not yet engaged in the HUB to obtain the required samples. When possible sample supply is identified, the biobank will receive a more detailed request form describing detailed requirements the context of the research program.

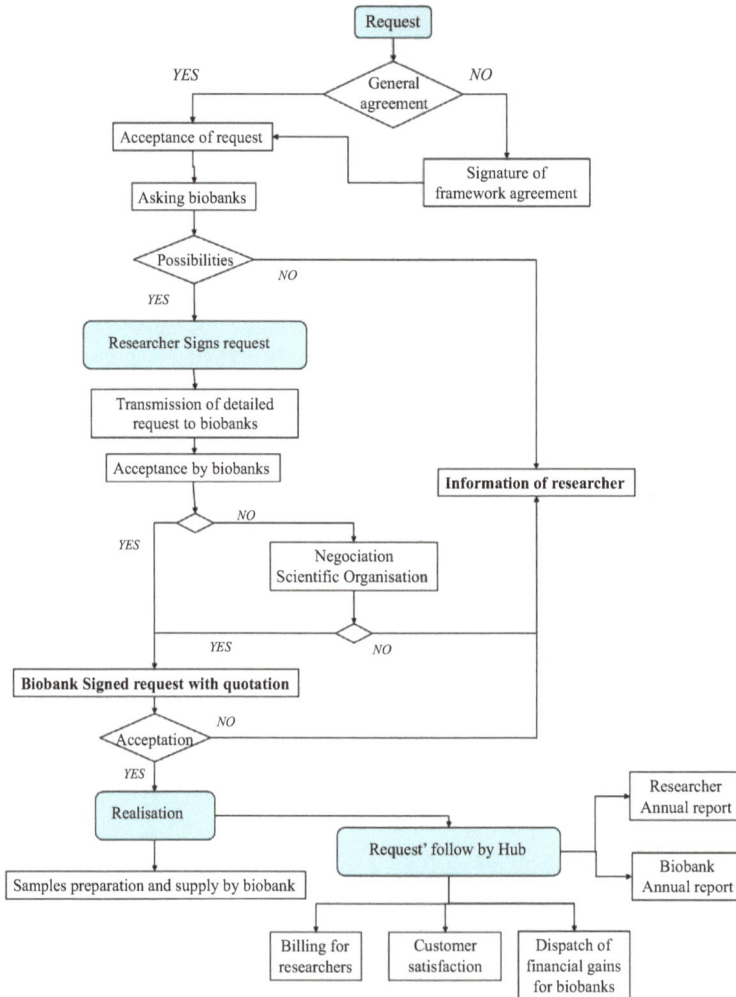

Fig. (2). Model of procedure concerning the workflow for a request treatment.

Using this information, biobanks can manage the request in accordance with their own procedures. The HUB only provides information about the possibility of sample distribution and does not interfere in the activities of the biobank. Its only requirement concerns the biobank's response time which must be under 10 days.

The first biobank responder is given priority to conclude the collaboration.

Acceptance by the biobanks is linked with a proposed quotation for services. If several biobanks are involved in a request, a common quotation proposed by HUB must be accepted by all biobanks before transmission to the research team.

The conclusion of each negotiation is represented by a request document signed by the principal researcher, the biobank director and the representative of HUB.

In accordance with the schedule defined, the biobank will supply the samples directly to the researcher's laboratory. The HUB does not centralize the samples before sending. This policy reduces the number of times that the samples are transported (which is often risky and costly) and assures transparent of movement of samples.

Invoices are exchanged as follows: The HUB sends an invoice to the researcher that covers both the quotation accepted by the biobank and fees for the administrative work of the HUB. Then in addition, the biobank issues an invoice to the HUB.

An additional role of HUB-BTB-3CR is to survey customer satisfaction and the performance of its organization to maintain continued improvement. Moreover, each participant in HUB-BTB-3CR receives an annual report to give them a global view of their participation.

CONCLUSION

Biobanks are becoming real partners of translational research besides fundamental and pharmaceutical research for the benefit of healthcare patients. To maintain their role and assure the management of biological resource collections in the long term they need to develop a sustainability policy. Different complementary solutions must be imagined. One of them is the development of sample sharing for pharmaceutical research under fee conditions.

Aware of economic and strategic issues of medical research, BioTech BANK and 3C-R have designed a new economic model for biobanking sustainability which links private research teams and biobanks in a win-win organization with the final objective of the better healthcare of patients.

As in the concept of circular economy [35] where the efficient use of resources creates economic, social and environmental value, the structuring of HUB-BT--3CR is based on an enhancement of flux of biological resources in favor of use rather than possession of property.

For academic biobanks,this provides a way to rethink the life cycle of biological resources to produce optimal results. As in a natural ecosystem, this model promotes a cycle of improvements: nothing is lost, all is used or reused.

Participation in HUB-BTB-3CR does not weaken scientific programs where biobanks are involved, but adds a complementary value to the collections with their use in pharmaceutical research. These public-private relationships are necessary to enhance translational research and develop beneficial treatments for patients [36] besides which they can become a significant source of financing.

The purpose of HUB-BTB-3CR is to accelerate scientific discovery, avoid loss of time for researchers, maximise sample use and to participate in the financial sustainability of biobanks. Based on the simplification of material transfer agreements and links between demand and supply, HUB-BTB-3CRcould represent an additional way to optimize the use of samples and obtain complementary financial support.

CONFLICT OF INTEREST

The authors confirm that they have no conflict of interest to declare for this publication.

ACKNOWLEDGEMENT

Declared none.

REFERENCES

[1]   OECD Best Practice Guidelines for Biological resource centres 2007.

[2]   ISBER Best practices for biorepositories: collection, storage, retrieval and distribution of biological materials for research. 3rd ed., 2011.

[3]   di Donato JH. Biobanking for rare for rare disease - Impact on personalised medecine. Advances in predictive, preventive and personalised medecine, Rare diseases - Integrative PPPM approach as the medecine of future. Springer 2014; Vol. 6: pp. 23-31.

[4]   Castillo-Pelayo T, Babinszky S, LeBlanc J, Watson PH. The importance of biobanking in cancer research. Biopreserv Biobank 2015; 13(3): 172-7.
       [http://dx.doi.org/10.1089/bio.2014.0061] [PMID: 26035006]

[5]   Zika E, Paci D, Schultein den Bäumen T, *et al.* Biobanks in Europe: Prospects for hamonisation and networking. Euromean Commission, Join Research Centre Institute for Porspective Technological Studies 2010.

[6]   Henderson GE, Cadigan RJ, Edwards TP, *et al.* Characterizing biobank organizations in the U.S: results from a national survey. Genome Med 2013; 5(1): 3.
       [http://dx.doi.org/10.1186/gm407] [PMID: 23351549]

[7]   Albert M, Bartlett J, Johnston RN, Schacter B, Watson P. Biobank bootstrapping: is biobank sustainability possible through cost recovery? Biopreserv Biobank 2014; 12(6): 374-80.
       [http://dx.doi.org/10.1089/bio.2014.0051] [PMID: 25496148]

[8]   Vaught J, Kelly A, Hewitt R. A review of international biobanks and networks: success factors and key benchmarks. Biopreserv Biobank 2009; 7(3): 143-50.
[http://dx.doi.org/10.1089/bio.2010.0003] [PMID: 24835880]

[9]   Anderlik M. Commercial biobanks and genetic research: ethical and legal issues. Am J Pharmacogenomics 2003; 3(3): 203-15.
[http://dx.doi.org/10.2165/00129785-200303030-00006] [PMID: 12814328]

[10]   Rogers J, Carolin T, Vaught J, Compton C. Biobankonomics: a taxonomy for evaluating the economic benefits of standardized centralized human biobanking for translational research. J Natl Cancer Inst Monogr 2011; 2011(42): 32-8.
[http://dx.doi.org/10.1093/jncimonographs/lgr010] [PMID: 21672893]

[11]   Simeon-Dubach D, Henderson MK. Sustainability in biobanking. Biopreserv Biobank 2014; 12(5): 287-91.
[http://dx.doi.org/10.1089/bio.2014.1251] [PMID: 25314050]

[12]   Turner A, Dallaire-Fortier C, Murtagh M. Biobank economics and the "commercialization problem". Spontaneous Generations: A journal for the History and Philosophy of Science 2013; 7(1): 69-80.

[13]   McDonald SA, Sommerkamp K, Egan-Palmer M, Kharasch K, Holtschlag V. Fee-for-service as a business model of growing importance: the academic biobank experience. Biopreserv Biobank 2012; 10(5): 421-5.
[http://dx.doi.org/10.1089/bio.2012.0017] [PMID: 23386922]

[14]   Parry-Jones A. Assessing the financial, operational, and social sustainability of a biobank: the Wales Cancer Bank case study. Biopreserv Biobank 2014; 12(6): 381-8. 203-215
[http://dx.doi.org/10.1089/bio.2014.0044]

[15]   Vaught J, Rogers J, Carolin T, Compton C. Biobankonomics: developing a sustainable business model approach for the formation of a human tissue biobank. J Natl Cancer Inst Monogr 2011; 2011(42): 24-31.
[http://dx.doi.org/10.1093/jncimonographs/lgr009] [PMID: 21672892]

[16]   Wilson GD, DAngelo K, Pruetz BL, Geddes TJ, Larson DM, Akervall J. The challenge of sustaining a hospital-based biobank and core molecular laboratory: the Beaumont experience. Biopreserv Biobank 2014; 12(5): 306-11.
[http://dx.doi.org/10.1089/bio.2014.0049] [PMID: 25314610]

[17]   Galli J, Oelrich J, Taussig MJ, Andreasson U, Ortega-Paino E, Landegren U. The Biobanking Analysis Resource Catalogue (BARCdb): a new research tool for the analysis of biobank samples. Nucleic Acids Res 2015; 43(Database issue): D1158-62.
[http://dx.doi.org/10.1093/nar/gku1008] [PMID: 25336620]

[18]   Verlinden M, Nys H, Ectors N, Huys I. Access to biobanks: harmonization across biobank initiatives. Biopreserv Biobank 2014; 12(6): 415-22.
[http://dx.doi.org/10.1089/bio.2014.0034] [PMID: 25496154]

[19]   Roessler BJ, Steneck NH, Connally L. The MICHR Genomic DNA BioLibrary: An empirical study of the ethics of biorepository development. J Empir Res Hum Res Ethics 2015; 10(1): 37-48.
[http://dx.doi.org/10.1177/1556264614564975] [PMID: 25742665]

[20]   Clément B, Yuille M, Zatloukal K, *et al.* Dagher G and the EU-US Expert Group on cost recovery in biobanks.Public biobanks: calculation and recovery of costs. Sc Trans Med 2014; 6(261).

[21]   Canadian Tissue Repository Network. Biospecimen User Fee Calculator: A comprehensive and easy to use tool that captures annual expenses, resources, and biospecimen accrual and calculates the appropriate user fees. Available from http://www.biobanking.org/webs/biobankcosting

[22]   Mora M, Angelini C, Bignami F, *et al.* The EuroBioBank Network: Ten years of hands-on experience of collaborative, transnational biobanking for rare diseases. Eur J Hum Genet 2014; 1-8.
[PMID: 25537360]

[23]   Carpenter JĖ, Clarke CL. Biobanking sustainabilityexperiences of the Australian Breast Cancer Tissue Bank (ABCTB). Biopreserv Biobank 2014; 12(6): 395-401.
[http://dx.doi.org/10.1089/bio.2014.0055] [PMID: 25496151]

[24]   Bravo E, Napolitano M, Santoro F, Belardelli F, Federic A. The Italian Hub of Population Biobanks as a potential tool for improving public health stewardship. Biopreserv Biobank 2013; 11(3): 173-5.
[http://dx.doi.org/10.1089/bio.2012.0064] [PMID: 23840926]

[25]   Virtual tumor bank of Canceropole GSO. Available from http://www.biobank-gso.org/apex/ f?p=200:1:1242380734223043

[26]   EuroBioBank catalogue. Available from http://www.eurobiobank.org/en/services/CatalogueHome .html

[27]   BBMRI catalogue. Available from http://bbmri-eric.eu/bbmri-eric-directory-2.0

[28]   Club 3C-R. Available from http://www.3cr-ressourcesbiologiques.com/ #!le-club-3cr-ressour-es-biologiques/c1sdk

[29]   Golubnitschaja O, Kinkorova J, Costigliola V. Predictive, preventive and personalised medicine as the hardcore of horizon 2020: EPMA position paper. EPMA J 2014; 5(1): 6.
[http://dx.doi.org/10.1186/1878-5085-5-6] [PMID: 24708704]

[30]   Rugnetta M, Whitney K. Paving the way for personalized medicine , 2009 [Access 25 Jan 2016]; Sci Prog. Available from http://www.scienceprogress.org/wp-content/uploads/2009/09/ personalized_ medicine.pdf

[31]   Liszewski K. Biobanking on Translational Omics. Bulging with molecular riches, next-generation biobanks plan to back personalized medicine. Gen 2015; 35(2)

[32]   Olson JE, Bielinski SJ, Ryu E, *et al.* Biobanks and personalized medicine. Clin Genet 2014; 86(1): 50-5.
[http://dx.doi.org/10.1111/cge.12370] [PMID: 24588254]

[33]   Bubela T, Guebert J, Mishra A. Use and misuse of material transfer agreements: lessons in proportionality from research, repositories, and litigation. PLoS Biol 2015; 13(2): e1002060.
[http://dx.doi.org/10.1371/journal.pbio.1002060] [PMID: 25646804]

[34]   Walsh JP, Cho C, Cohen WM. Patents, material transfers and access to research inputs in biomedical research 2005.

[35]   Ellen MacArthur Foundation and McKinsey&Company. Towards the circular economy: Accelerating the scale-up across global supply chains 2014. World Economic Forum. Available from http://www3.weforum.org/docs/WEF_ENV_TowardsCircularEconomy_Report_2014.pdf

[36]   Hofman P, Bréchot C, Zatloukal K, Dagher G, Clément B. Public-private relationships in biobanking: a still underestimated key component of open innovation. Virchows Arch 2014; 464(1): 3-9.
[http://dx.doi.org/10.1007/s00428-013-1524-z] [PMID: 24337181]

SUBJECT INDEX

Elena Salvaterra and Julie Corfield (Eds.)
All rights reserved-© 2017 Bentham Science Publishers

www.ingramcontent.com/pod-product-compliance
Lightning Source LLC
Chambersburg PA
CBHW041729210326
41598CB00008B/827

* 9 7 8 1 6 8 1 0 8 5 1 1 1 *